>1 C
is TOO MANY!

Join us in our goal to decrease the number of falls in older adults.

Download **free resources** at www.thebookofbalance.com/resources

*More than **one out of four** older adults fall each year, and those who fall once are 2 to 3 times more likely to fall again.[1,2]

1. Stevens JA, Ballesteros MF, Mack KA, Rudd RA, DeCaro E, Adler G. Gender differences in seeking care for falls in the aged   Medicare Population. Am J Prev Med 2012;43: 59–62.
2. O'Loughlin J et al. Incidence of and risk factors for falls and injurious falls among the community-dwelling elderly. American journal of epidemiology, 1993, 137:342-54

THE BOOK OF
BALANCE

REHAB SECRETS TO IMPROVE YOUR BALANCE
AND DECREASE YOUR RISK OF FALLING

LEX GONZALES, PT, DPT

Text © 2018 by Lex Gonzales, PT, DPT
Illustrations by Jonathan Edwards

Printed in the United States of America

ISBN- book - 9781985646483
ISBN- ebook – 198564648X

This book is dedicated
to all those who ceased to be my patients...
and became my friends.

TABLE OF CONTENTS

ABOUT THIS BOOK

"We cannot change what we are not aware of, and once we are aware, we cannot help but change."
- Sheryl Sandberg

This book is not an academic treatise, though you can go deeper into the academic research and science by considering the citations and bibliography I listed in this book. Rather, the goal of this book is to help you improve your balance and decrease your risk of falling through the judicious application of the knowledge and skills you will learn from its pages.

This book is not for those who only *like to know*. This book is for those who *want to do*. To improve your balance and decrease your risk of falling, you must act on the information you learned. Contrary to what Francis Bacon said in 1620, knowledge is not always power. Implemented knowledge is.

Don't read this book.
Consume it. Study it. Implement it.

As early as 2006, the Centers for Disease Control and Prevention (CDC) and the National Center for Injury Prevention and Control (NCIPC) has identified Fall Prevention as a priority. Yet, despite evidence from countless studies supporting the beneficial effects of a fall reduction and balance program, there is still a lack of discussion between healthcare practitioners and patients on this topic. Imagine what could be saved in terms of physical, emotional, psychological, or financial costs if the discussion, screening, and intervention happens BEFORE a patient suffers a fall.

Oftentimes, physical therapists end up treating the *result* of a fall, not the *cause,* i.e. we treat the hip fracture after a fall, not what *caused* the fall.

I always believed that the more my patients know about their condition, the better able they are in helping themselves. I've seen the veracity of that belief in my clinical practice – the more I teach my patients about their health, the more empowered they are in taking care of themselves. The more they know, the healthier they become.

That is my compelling mission with this book.

Though this book will address most general concerns related to balance and the risks of falling, every person will have different contributing factors specific to himself or herself that will affect them differently. I recommend that you consult your physical therapist or physician to get an individualized evaluation and assessment BEFORE starting the exercise program I outline in this book.

Falling is not a result nor is it a compulsory companion of aging. A review of numerous fall intervention studies has established strong evidence that fall prevention and balance programs can reduce falls. This book will provide you with information on the many factors putting you at risk of falling and the multi-component intervention you can implement to address those risk factors.

Let us work together to improve your balance.

Together, let us decrease the number of falls in older adults.

Lex Gonzales, PT, DPT

INTRODUCTION

"An ounce of prevention is worth a pound of cure."
- Benjamin Franklin

WHEN is the best time to work on improving your balance?

Before you have a fall!

When is the second-best time to work on improving your balance?

Before you have another fall!

Studies have shown that having sustained a fall increases a person's risk of sustaining another fall. [1, 2] Even without a resulting injury from a fall, some people develop a fear of falling that may limit their daily activities. [3]

In fact, fear of falling is so prevalent in community-dwelling older adults that it is has been identified as an independent risk factor for reduced quality of life. [4] Once a person becomes fearful of performing simple daily activities, they avoid more

---

[1] Vellas B, Wayne S, Romero L, Baumgartner R, Garry P. Fear of falling and restriction of mobility in elderly fallers. Age and Ageing 1997;26:189-193
[2] A report of the Kellogg International Working Group on the prevention of falls by the elderly. The prevention of falls in later life. Dan Med Bull 1987 34 Suppl 4:1-24
[3] Tinetti M et al. Fear of falling and fall-related efficacy in relationship to functioning among community-living elders. Journal of gerontology, 1994, 49:M140-M147.
[4] T. Hadjistavropoulos, K. Delbaere, T.D. Fitzgerald Reconceptualizing the role of fear of falling and balance confidence in fall risk J Aging Health, 23 (1) (2011), pp. 3-23

challenging movements or strenuous activities. This self-imposed limitation in activity level leads to reduced mobility, a decline in strength and physical fitness, and decreased independence.[5]

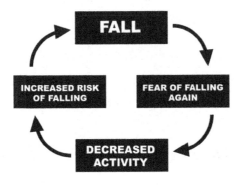

The Fall Cycle

The diagram above represents the vicious cycle of falls: Sustaining a fall results in an increased *fear* of falling. Fear of falling, in turn, results in a self-imposed decrease in activity. Finally, because of declining strength and physical fitness from decreased activity, an *actual* risk of falling develops. This fall cycle perpetuates a negative impact on the quality of life of an individual following a fall.

The concept of the fall cycle reminds me of my patient Betsy*. Betsy is a dainty 66-year-old lady with the mental sharpness and energy of a 40-year-old. Her favorite thing to do is playing with her grandchildren - all 7 of them!

She told me how one day her daughter and son-in-law had asked her to watch over their two-year-old son as they had to leave for an emergency business meeting.

---

[5] Zijlstra GA, van Haastregt JC, van Rossum E, et al. Interventions to reduce fear of falling in community-living older people: a systematic review. J Am Geriatr Soc 2007;55(4):603-615

Betsy was not only able to keep up with the boundless energy of her toddler grandson, she wished that her daughter and son-in-law would have extended their business meeting so she could have spent more time running after her grandson.

That is my definition of "aging backward!"

Unfortunately, Betsy's zest for life changed one fateful morning.

As she would normally do every morning, Betsy walked out to her driveway to pick up her morning paper. As Betsy stooped down to grab the newspaper from the ground, she lost her balance. In her attempt to catch her balance, Betsy slipped and fell on her side.

She immediately felt a sharp, excruciating pain in her left hip. Betsy tried to get up but the pain on her hip was so severe, she could barely move without aggravating it. She lay down on her driveway writhing in pain until her neighbor found her and called emergency ambulance services. A full 3 hours after she fell!

Betsy broke her left hip when she fell. Though she eventually recovered from her surgery and went home after hip rehabilitation, Betsy was so traumatized by her experience that she refrained from playing with her grandchildren. She was afraid of falling.

Betsy was at this state of underlying fear when I first worked with her. She has cut back on her activities so much that she has lost her energy, her strength, and her balance. Her children brought her to me looking for answers. They were worried that she had lost her zest for life. Gone were the boundless energy and mental sharpness her family and friends knew her for.

Without proper evaluation of the patient, friends or family members may attribute this decline in physical activity or lack of social engagement as a natural part of aging. Often, the underlying reason a lot of older adults withdraw from or limit their activities of daily living is because of their fear of falling, not their age.

When Betsy started, she was unsure of her balance faculties and less trusting of the balance program I formulated for her. As she was not certain of her ability to keep herself from falling, I started her program with less-challenging exercises. She started her balance training program in a sitting position! Doing so allowed Betsy to work on improving her balance skills at a level she was comfortable with. More importantly, it allowed her to develop her confidence knowing that she could build up the skills she learned from one level to the next.

And she did.

By the time Betsy completed her balance program, she was walking independently without the aid of a walker or a cane.

The best part? Betsy welcomed back the company of her grandchildren!

This book is about how Betsy and I (and several other patients you will meet in this book) worked together to improve her balance, break free from her fear of falling, and live independently with vigor again.

In the words of Betsy, *"This balance program gave me back my life."*

*To protect patient privacy and confidentiality, names have been changed; in some cases, several people have been condensed into one to make a clearer point.

PART 1

CHAPTER 1

WHAT IS BALANCE?

"Life is like riding a bicycle. To keep your balance, you must keep moving."
- Albert Einstein

The word *balance* first meant, "An instrument used to weigh things." It traces its origin from two Latin words, *bi*, meaning twice or having two, and *lanx*, meaning scale pan. [1] As trade and commerce blossomed in the ancient times, merchants started exchanging their goods for precious stones and metals; a practice commonly known as bartering. When the volume of goods being exchanged grew, the task of counting irregularly shaped precious stones and metals by the pieces became increasingly laborious and inefficient. Merchants needed a way to assess the value of their goods without spending too much time in counting

> **bartering ~** trading or exchanging services or goods for other services or goods with no money involved.

---

[1] https://www.merriam-webster.com/dictionary/balance, Accessed February 27, 2017

stones and metals. Out of this necessity, weighing scales were born.

The first weighing scales were called *balances*. These were two scale pans attached to an overhead beam fixed on a pole. The merchants measure the value of their goods by weighing it on one pan against the weight of the precious stones or metals placed on the other pan. Once equilibrium or balance is reached between the two scale pans, the value of the goods sold is determined.

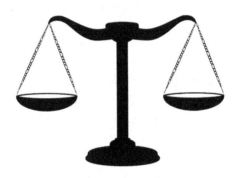

bal•ance /baləns/[1]

: *an instrument for weighing*
: *a means of judging or deciding*
: *an aesthetically pleasing integration of element*
: *stability produced by even distribution of weight*
  on each side of the vertical axis
: *mental and emotional steadiness*
: *physical equilibrium*

center of mass ~ a point at the center of your total body mass.

Much like the weighing scale, your body's center of mass (the pole in the middle of the scale) must be maintained within your base of support for you to maintain a stable upright position.

According to Dr. Mary Tinetti, Director of the Yale Program on Aging, and a pioneer in the study of morbidity due to falls by elderly people, "There is a physiological definition of balance which incorporates proprioception, vision, and other components that clinicians tend to agree on. But there also is a functional definition of balance that refers to the ability to change positions, maneuver through the environment, and withstand perturbations, which clinicians don't always agree."

base of support ~ the area beneath a person that includes every point of contact that the person makes with the supporting surface.

It is hard to educate patients if we, healthcare professionals, cannot agree on a definition of balance. My patients do not come to me asking for a complex definition of balance. They just want to know how they can improve their balance so they can keep themselves from falling. A simpler definition of balance you and I will use in the context of this book is, *"The ability to have your weight spread within the limits of your base of support so that you do not fall."*

For you to maintain your balance, you should be able to keep your body's weight and center of mass within your base of support. That is true whether your body is moving or stationary. The second (it takes less than a minute) your body weight is displaced outside your base of support, you risk "tipping the scale" and losing your balance.

Much like the weighing scale used in the olden times, if one or several systems of your body is deficient, you will be tipping the scale toward imbalance. As the human body ages, there are several age-associated body systems changes that tip the scale toward imbalance. Being aware of these age-associated changes is the first step toward finding solutions to your balance problems. It enables you to take the necessary steps toward improving or compensating for the body systems that have declined with age.

Even though I wrote this book using as little medical jargon as possible to help every reader understand the intricacies of balance, there are a few terms specific to the study of balance that, once understood clearly, can be applied more appropriately to your own situation.

anticipatory postural control ~ prepared or pre-programmed response to maintain stability.

One important terminology commonly used in the study of balance is **proactive or anticipatory postural control**. These are the actions you plan in anticipation of challenges or disturbances to your balance.

Faced with a puddle of water in a walkway, you anticipate taking a bigger step, or maybe even a hop, to avoid getting your shoes wet. Whatever you did, you already planned, or anticipated, how to keep your weight within your base of support to keep your balance.

reactive postural control ~ modified response to an external disturbance or environmental demand.

In contrast, when faced with an unexpected challenge to your balance, you respond with **compensatory or reactive postural control**. An example would be when you are suddenly bumped while walking, or when your foot slips after stepping on a banana peel. You keep yourself from falling by "catching", or compensating, for your balance.

Whereas anticipatory postural control strategies can be planned, reactive postural control strategies are unplanned, often quick and reflexive actions. As these two postural control strategies require different responses, it is important that an exercise program is designed toward improving both.

postural control strategies ~ a plan of action meant to achieve, maintain, or restore a state of balance during any posture or activity.

Moreover, there are at least three postural control strategies that are commonly used to maintain your balance.

To better understand these concepts, you can try each one while reading this book.

First, you will try the **ankle strategy** by reading this book in a standing position. As you are reading this book while standing, you are subconsciously contracting the muscles surrounding your ankles to keep your body upright. You keep your body upright by controlling to a minimum how much your body sways. In the ankle strategy, your upper and lower body move as a single entity about your ankle joint.

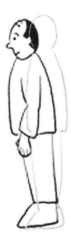

Ankle Strategy

Next, while still standing, try reaching for an object about 10-12 inches away from you without moving your feet. As you are reaching away from you, notice that you are bending about your hip joint. You just kept your balance by using the **hip strategy**. In the hip strategy, your upper and lower body move in opposite directions. This is an important strategy to use when your body needs to sway more to keep your balance.

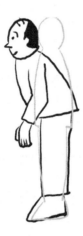

Hip Strategy

Finally, when the object you are trying to reach is beyond the limits of your stability, you will need to take a step to reach the object without losing your balance. That is called the **step strategy**. You use the step strategy whenever you need to establish a new base of support in order not to fall.

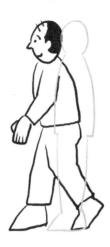

Step Strategy

Traditionally, balance training programs often utilize **single-task** conditions or exercises. Single-task training means that you are practicing functional activities requiring balance in isolation.[2] These are the exercises you do while you focus on just one task at a time. Single-task training is important in laying the groundwork or foundation for improving your balance. However, single-task training may not translate to balance requirements needed under real-world situations.

Most activities you do every day often require you to maintain your balance while you are doing two or more tasks at the same time. You may be standing on a sidewalk while looking around at the road signs at the same time. You may be walking while talking on the phone. Most often than not, you will find yourself doing more than one thing at any given time. These conditions are called **dual-task** or divided- attention tasks.

---

[2] Silsupadol P, Siu KC, Shumway-Cook A. Training of balance under single- and dual-task conditions in older adults with balance impairment. Phys Ther. 2006;269-281

Dual-task training occurs when 2 or more activities are performed simultaneously.[3]

Performance of tasks requiring your divided attention results in decreased postural control and increased instability in walking – both resulting in an increased risk of falling.

Balance training under both single- and dual-task conditions are necessary not only to improve your balance and decrease your risk of falling, but also to optimize your independence in performing the activities you would normally do every day.

What does the research say?

A systematic review and meta-analyses of multiple randomized clinical trials related to balance found that the most effective intervention for reducing the risk of falling involves a multifactorial assessment and management.[4]

Strategies that combine interventions addressing more than one risk factor, including "multidisciplinary, multifactorial, health/environmental risk factor screening, and intervention programs" significantly reduced the number of participants falling and reduced the incidence of falls among community-dwelling older people.[5]

A 2004 report evaluated multiple studies, and the resulting analysis demonstrated that multiple intervention programs are more effective than exercise alone. The authors concluded

---

[3] Plummer P, Villalobos R, Vayda M, Moser M, Johnson E. Feasibility of dual-task gait training for community-dwelling adults after stroke: a case series. Stroke Research and Treatment. Vol.2014; Art.538602
[4] Chang JT, Morton SC, Rubenstein LZ, Mojica WA, Maglione M, Suttorp MJ, et al. Interventions for the prevention of falls in older adults: systematic review and meta-analysis of randomized clinical trials. *BMJ*. 2004; 328:680
[5] Gillespie, L.D. et al (2004) Interventions for Preventing Falls in Elderly People (Cochrane Review). The Cochrane Library, Issue 2.

that multiple intervention strategies were particularly effective for fall prevention.[6]

Whereas a lot of balance programs focus on one component of balance and call it a balance program (i.e. strengthening exercises only, visual-vestibular exercises only, home modification only, etc.), this book will provide you with information on the multiple factors and components that play a role in improving your balance and decreasing your risk of falling.

In Part 1 of The Book of Balance, you will learn about these many factors that contribute to your balance and risk of falling. Use this information to discuss with your physical therapist or physician specific areas that apply to your own situation and to tailor your intervention accordingly.

In Part 2 of The Book of Balance, you will find exercises designed to improve your strength, flexibility, posture, multisensory function, coordination, reaction time, and balance strategies. Use these to improve your balance and decrease your risk of falling.

Having learned the definition and application of each, give special emphasis to those areas you feel you need to improve the most to *balance* the scale!

---

[6] Weatherall, M. (2004) Prevention of falls and fall-related fractures in community-dwelling older adults: a meta-analysis of estimates of effectiveness based on recent guidelines. Internal Medicine Journal; 34: 3, 102–108.

CHAPTER 2

LET US BEGIN WITH THE BASICS – OUR ABC'S AND TUG'S

"To begin with the end in mind means to start with a clear understanding of your destination. It means to know where you're going so that you better understand where you are now and so that the steps you take are always in the right direction."
- Stephen Covey

To know where you are going, you first must know where you are standing right now.

How is your balance today?

If you were to walk around your house now; through all the narrow or dimly-lit hallways, on fluffy carpet or cold tile, walk up or down stairs, step over to get in your bathtub or shower, or walk outside on an uneven driveway; how confident are you that your balance will not betray you?

I asked my friend Edward these questions, and his reply to me was, "I don't really think about these things until I'm there already." It may be hard to believe, but Edward's answer is a typical response I get from a lot of my patients. We tend to not think about nor consider these obstacles until these obstacles confront us.

To measure how much your balance has improved, you first need to know how good (or bad) your balance is today and compare it with your balance after applying the lessons and exercises you will learn from this book. You need to have baseline data to compare your progress after completing the balance program outlined in this book.

There is a battery of tests and measures that physical therapists and physicians utilize to test a patient's balance. Since I cannot hold you by the hand, we will utilize a self-administered balance questionnaire[1] and an easy to perform test with excellent reliability when performed among older adults.[2] These tests will give you a baseline score that you can then compare after you follow all the lessons and strategies you find in this book.

The balance questionnaire we will be using is called Activities-specific Balance Confidence (ABC) Scale. This questionnaire has been shown to be a valid and reliable measure for the assessment of balance confidence among community-dwelling

---

[1] Powell LE & Myers AM. The Activities-specific Balance Confidence (ABC) Scale. Journal of Gerontology Med Sci 1995; 50(1):M28-34.
[2] Nordin, E., Rosendahl, E., et al. (2006). "Timed "Up & Go" test: reliability in older people dependent in activities of daily living--focus on cognitive state." Phys Ther 86(16649889): 646-655.

older adults and is literally as easy to answer as its acronym, ABC![3]

There are 16 questions, corresponding to different activities you would normally do on an average day. For each of the questions, you will indicate your level of confidence in performing that activity without losing your balance or becoming unsteady.

You will score yourself on a scale from 0% (*No confidence*) to 100% (*Completely Confident*). There are no right or wrong answers, so be honest with yourself when answering the questions. Only you will benefit the most with your answers.

I have included a copy of this test below, but if you want a larger typeset that will be easier to read in one piece of paper, you can download and print a copy of this test from www.thebookofbalance.com/resources

The Activities-specific Balance Confidence (ABC) Scale

Instructions:

For each of the following activities, please indicate your level of confidence in doing the activity without losing your balance or becoming unsteady by choosing one of the percentage points on the scale from 0% to 100%

If you do not currently do the activity in question, try and imagine how confident you would be if you had to do the activity.

---

[3] Filiatraut J, Gauvin L, et al. Evidence of the psychometric qualities of a simplified version of the Activities-specific Balance Confidence Scale for community dwelling seniors. Archives of Physical Medicine and Rehabilitation 88(5):664-672

If you normally use a walking aid to do the activity or hold onto someone, rate your confidence as if you were using these supports.

0% 10 20 30 40 50 60 70 80 90 100%
No Confidence   Completely Confident

How confident are you that you will not lose your balance or become unsteady when you...

1. walk around the house?   _____%

2. walk up or down stairs?   _____%

3. bend over and pick up a slipper from the front of a closet floor?   _____%

4. reach for a small can off a shelf at eye level?   _____%

5. stand on your tip toes and reach for something above your head?   _____%

6. stand on a chair and reach for something?   _____%

7. sweep the floor?   _____%

8. walk outside the house to a car parked in the driveway?   _____%

9. get into or out of a car?   _____%

10. walk across a parking lot to the mall?   _____%

11. walk up or down a ramp?   _____%

12. walk in a crowded mall where people rapidly walk past you?   _____%

13. are bumped into by people as you walk through the mall?   _____%

14. step onto or off an escalator while you are holding onto a railing?   _____%

15. step onto or off an escalator while holding parcels in such a way that you cannot hold onto the railing?   _____%

16. walk outside on icy sidewalks? _____%

TOTAL SCORE: _____

DATE: _____

To get your ABC score, add all your ratings (possible range of 0 to 1600) and divide by 16.

Reference Values[4]

>80% - high level of physical functioning
50%-80% - moderate level of physical functioning
<50% - low level of physical functioning

Another test we will perform is called the Timed Up and Go or TUG Test. This test is a fast and reliable diagnostic tool. The result of this test correlates with your walking speed, balance, and functional level. A normal, healthy older adult usually completes the task in ten seconds or less. A very frail or weak, elderly adult with poor mobility may take 2 minutes or even longer.[5,6] Log in to www.thebookofbalance.com/resources to download and print the TUG test.

Timed Up and Go (TUG)

General Instructions:

1. Have another person monitor a watch or timer for you.
2. Begin the test by sitting correctly (hips all the way to the back of the seat) in a chair with armrests. The chair

---

[4] Myers AM, Fletcher PC, Myers AN, Sherk W. Discriminative and evaluative properties of the ABC Scale. J Gerontology A Biol Sci Med Sci. 1998;53:M287-M294.
[5] Bohannon RW. Reference values for the Timed Up and Go Test: A Descriptive Meta-Analysis. Journal of Geriatric Physical Therapy, 2006;29(2):64-8.
[6] Shumway-Cook A, Brauer S, Woollacott M. Predicting the probability for falls in community-dwelling older adults using the timed up & go test. Phys Ther. 2000;80:896-903.

should be stable and positioned so that it will not move when you move from sitting to standing.

3. You can use the armrests during the sit to stand and stand to sit movements.
4. Place a piece of tape or another marker on the floor 3 meters (9.84 feet) away from the chair.

Test Instructions:

1. On the word GO, you will stand up, walk to the marker on the floor, turn around, and walk back to the chair and sit down. Walk at your regular pace.
2. The person monitoring the timer should start timing on the word "GO" and stop timing when you are seated again correctly in the chair with your back resting against the back of the chair.
3. You should wear your regular footwear and may use any gait aid (cane, walker, etc.) that you normally use during ambulation, but you may not be assisted by another person.
4. There is no time limit. You may stop and rest (but not sit down) if you need to.

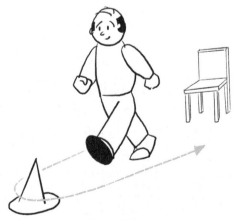

TUG Test

Normative Reference Values by Age

Age Group	Time in Seconds (95% Confidence Interval)
60 – 69 years	8.1 (7.1 – 9.0)
70 – 79 years	9.2 (8.2 – 10.2)
80 – 99 years	11.3 (10.0 – 12.7)

Cut-off Values Predictive of Falls

Group	Time in Second
1. Community-Dwelling Frail Older Adults	> 14 associated with high fall risk
2. Post-op hip fracture patients at time of discharge	> 24 predictive of falls within 6 months after hip fracture
3. Frail older adults	> 30 predictive of requiring assistive device for ambulation and being dependent on ADLs

ACTION STEP

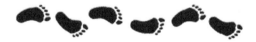

✓ Download and print a copy of the ABC Scale and TUG Test from www.thebookofbalance.com/resources to get a larger typeset version on a single piece of paper that will be easier to read. Post the results on your refrigerator (or anywhere you can easily see and access).

Tip: We will do this test again after you finish your balance program, so hold on to it!

CHAPTER 3

KNOW WHAT CAUSES YOU TO FALL

"If you know the enemy and know yourself,
you need not fear the result of a hundred battles."
- Sun Tzu

EXTRINSIC and INTRINSIC CAUSES

ON his first visit, my patient Paul and his wife Martha were arguing as they tried to explain the cause of his frequent falls. Martha argued that something was wrong with Paul's balance that caused him to fall more than three times in one month. She contended that Paul was just being proud by declaring that nothing is wrong with himself.

Mid-sentence, Paul interrupted Martha and passionately argued that it is their poorly-lit stairway, and a hallway filled with Martha's cats that caused him to fall. As he gets up in the morning and staggers toward the kitchen, Paul explained that walking down the poorly lighted stairs and walking in the hallway while thinking of Martha's cats is akin to walking blindfolded while trying to evade landmines.

I know. Only husbands can think of such colorful analogies!

The truth is, Paul's falls can be explained in between both arguments[1,2].

spatial orientation ~ being able to change location in space in relation to objects you can see.	Paul's declining vision affects his spatial orientation. The dimly-lit hallway compounds the challenge of orienting himself relative to the location of Martha's cats. Paul is right in comparing it to landmines!

The landmines that Paul refers to are called the extrinsic (or external) reasons for falls. Extrinsic causes of falls include environmental hazards, medications, visual and environmental conditions, and even poor footwear.

Paul's declining vision that Martha refers to is called intrinsic (or internal) reason for falls. Intrinsic causes of falls include poor vision, deteriorating vestibular system, poor posture, reduced physical activity, presence of multiple medical conditions, and cognitive or psychological reasons.

To find solutions to your balance problems, it is important that you identify both intrinsic and extrinsic reasons that may increase your risk of falling.

[1] Blake AJ, Morgan K, Bendall MJ, Dal-losso H, et al. Falls by elderly people at home: prevalence and associated risk factors. Age and Ageing 1988;17:365-372
[2] Rubenstein L, Josephson K. Falls and their prevention in the elderly people: what does the evidence show? Med Clin N Am 2006;90:807-824

In the following chapters, I will help you identify these intrinsic and extrinsic factors. Right now, I would like you to think of the possible reasons or factors that may affect your balance or put you at risk of falling.

Writing the reasons down on paper will help you identify the different factors that you and I can focus on to improve your balance.

Extrinsic (external) Factors	Intrinsic (internal) Factors

ACTION STEP

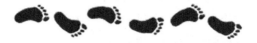

- ✓ Fill in the box with the different reasons or factors that you think may affect your balance or increase your risk of falling.

CHAPTER 4

EXTRINSIC RISK FACTORS

"You cannot control what happens to you, but you can control your attitude toward what happens to you, and in that, you will be mastering change rather than allowing it to master you."
– Brian Tracy

I learn a lot from my collaborative work with occupational therapy practitioners. They are the experts in identifying and eliminating environmental barriers to a patient's independence.

occupational therapist ~ licensed professionals who help people across the lifespan participate in the things they want and need to do through the therapeutic use of everyday activities (ADL).[6]

To improve a person's engagement with their environment and increase their independence in the performance of their activities of daily living (ADL), occupational therapists look at adaptations to the environment or modifications to the performance of a person's ADL.

While working with Paul, I asked my occupational therapist colleague to look further into the extrinsic factors that may have contributed to increasing Paul's risk of falling. She interviewed Paul and Martha, and the list she came up with bewildered both.

activities of daily living (ADL) ~ things you normally do in daily living including any daily activity you perform for self-care such as feeding, bathing, dressing, grooming, work, homemaking, and leisure.

Paul and Martha acknowledged that the list was an eye-opener. The occupational therapist listed common and mundane things that Paul and Martha see every day. In fact, they see them so often, they ceased to notice or pay attention to them. After reading the list, both exclaimed, "Why didn't we think of that?"

I expanded the list below, and as you peruse it, check the items that are already in good condition and do not need modification and work on checking off the items that need to be addressed.

Extrinsic Risk Factors at Home

GOOD   BAD

HOME ACCESS:
1. Level walkways with no cracks, holes, or gaps
2. Raised thresholds
3. Easily managed door knobs and locks
4. Non-slippery outdoor steps
5. Secure hand railings
6. Well-lit entrance

FLOOR SURFACES:
1. Loose rugs with crimp edges
2. Slippery floors in the kitchen, shower, or bathroom
3. Uneven surfaces, cracks in the floor, or floors that are buckling
4. Cluttered books, magazines, toys, etc. on the floor
5. Cords and wires on the floor
6. Stairs in poor repair or uneven steps
7. Stairs with loose or no handrails
8. Non-slip mat by your kitchen sink
9. Clear access to bathroom, bedroom, kitchen, and living areas

FURNITURE:
1. Low-lying furniture that obstructs your way
2. Cabinet shelves too high or too low
3. Beds too high or too low
4. Chairs that have armrests that you can push up from
5. Unstable chair or table that cannot support your weight
6. Frequently used items stored within your reach

BATHROOM:
1. Grab bars in bathtub or shower
2. Grab bars by the toilet
3. Low toilet seats
4. Non-slip mats by your bathroom sink, bathtub, or shower

STAIRWAY:
1. Outline and edge of each step clearly seen
2. Secure hand railings
3. Carpets or runners fastened down
4. Adequate lighting

LIGHTING:
1. Night lights in the bedroom, stairwells, hallways, and living areas
2. Flashlight by your bed
3. Burned-out light bulbs
4. Glare from windows and artificial lighting
5. Adequate lighting in the stairways and hallways

OTHER:
1. Loose or ill-fitting shoes (flip-flops and high-heeled shoes are notorious)
2. Hard to reach phones
3. Inappropriate or ill-measured walking aids and equipment
4. No designated area for pets
5. Wheelchair or rolling walker with dysfunctional brakes

Another often-overlooked extrinsic factor consistently associated with risk for falls is the role of medications.

I first saw Barry in a skilled nursing and rehabilitation facility where he was admitted after staying in a hospital for 7 days. His wife brought him to the hospital after he became progressively weak over several days. He was diagnosed as having pneumonia and was so weak he stayed in bed for most of the time he was in the hospital.

vital signs ~ clinical measurements that indicate the state of a patient's essential body functions.

While his vital signs (i.e. blood pressure, pulse rate, respiratory rate, etc.) were being monitored in the hospital, they noticed that his blood pressure was unusually high. He was referred to a cardiologist and was prescribed a hypertension medication to control his blood

34

pressure. Barry continued to take the hypertension medication when I started working with him at the skilled nursing and rehabilitation facility.

When I started my evaluation, I checked Barry's blood pressure while he was laying down in bed. Seeing that his blood pressure was normal, I proceeded to ask Barry to get up from the bed to assess how much assistance he would need.

cardiologist ~ a doctor who specializes in the study and treatment of heart disease and heart abnormalities.

Barry could get up into a standing position by himself, but after standing for a few minutes, he reported feeling lightheaded and clammy. I had Barry lie back down with his head flat on the bed. After a few minutes, Barry reported feeling back to normal again.

When I asked him if it was his first time he'd had that experience, Barry replied, "I've had these feeling like I'm about to pass out on several occasions; especially when I first get up in the morning."

After 5 minutes of lying down in bed, I checked Barry's blood pressure again. Again, his blood pressure was within the normal limits for his age.

orthostatic hypotension ~ a form of low blood pressure that happens when you stand up from sitting or lying down.

I explained to Barry that I suspect he was having an orthostatic hypotension and that I would be measuring his orthostatic blood pressure.

To measure orthostatic blood

pressure, you should check your blood pressure in three positions:

1. First, when you are lying down (for at least 5 minutes).
2. Second, when you change position to sitting or standing.
3. Finally, after about 3 minutes of sitting or standing.

A decrease of more than 20mm Hg in **systolic** *or more than 10 mm Hg in* **diastolic** *blood pressure after 3 minutes of sitting or standing is indicative of orthostatic hypotension.*

systolic pressure ~ the top number in your blood pressure; refers to the amount of pressure in your arteries during contraction of your heart muscle.

Barry's blood pressure while laying down in bed was 120/80 mm Hg. After standing for about 3 minutes, his blood pressure dropped to 90/60 mm Hg. No wonder Barry got lightheaded and clammy every time he stood up; he was experiencing orthostatic hypotension!

I taught Barry a simple technique to help decrease the symptoms of orthostatic hypotension and decrease his risk of falling each time he got up. Before he

diastolic pressure ~ the bottom number in your blood pressure; refers to the minimum arterial pressure during relaxation of your heart muscles.

changed his position from lying to sitting or from sitting to standing, I asked Barry to first do 10-15 repetitions of ankle pump exercises. This exercise assists the heart in circulating blood flow from the legs. As he assumes the new position, I

also asked him to stay still and breathe deeply for 30 seconds, or until the lightheadedness disappears, before moving any further.

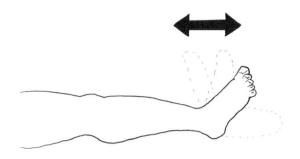

Ankle Pump Exercise

After my evaluation, I discussed my findings with Barry's physician, and the physician proceeded to adjust the dosage of the blood pressure medication Barry was taking.

Since the adjustment of his medication, Barry has been able to participate in standing activities without experiencing any lightheadedness or dizziness. It gave him confidence that he can stand up and walk without fear of falling.

Another risk factor for falling related to medications is polypharmacy. Polypharmacy is defined as the concurrent use of 4 or more medications. If you have several chronic diseases, i.e. high blood pressure, diabetes, high cholesterol, etc., chances are, you may be taking several medications intended to address each of those chronic disease conditions. The different intended effects of the medications you are taking, coupled with the interactions between those medications, may have an adverse effect on your balance. The use of four or more medications is associated with a nine-fold increased risk of cognitive impairment and fear of falling.[1]

---

[1] Todd C, Skelton D. (2004) What are the main risk factors for falls among older people and what are the most effective interventions to prevent these falls? Copenhagen, WHO Regional Office for Europe (Health Evidence Network report; http://www.euro.who.int/document/E82552.pdf, accessed 5 April 2004)

Also, if you are taking medications intended to affect your mind, behavior, or emotions, i.e. depression, sedation, anxiety, etc. (psychotropic medications), your risk of falling increases.[2]

Check the label of the medications you are currently taking to see if they have side effects that include dizziness, confusion, or fatigue.

The direct and side effects of the medications you are taking should be considered as you do an inventory of the extrinsic risk factors that may put you at a higher risk of falling.

Ask your physician to review all your medications and to minimize or withdraw, if appropriate, medications that put you at a high risk of falling.[3]

As you have seen, the extrinsic risk factors for falls at home and the role of medications are factors that can be easily fixed or modified. Some studies found that extrinsic risk factors account for 30%-50% of falls.[4,5]

For this chapter's ACTION STEP, look at the list again and fix or modify the items that need to be corrected. Also, ask your physician to review, and adjust as necessary, the medications you are currently taking.

---

[2] Leipzig RM1, Cumming RG, Tinetti ME, Drugs and falls in older people: a systematic review and meta-analysis I. Psychotropic drugs, J Am Geriatr Soc. 47(1),1999,30-9.

[3] Campbell, A. J., Robertson, M. C., Gardner, M. M., Norton, R. N., & Buchner, D. M. (1999). Psychotropic medication withdrawal and a home-based exercise program to prevent falls: A randomized, controlled trial. *Journal of the American Geriatrics Society, 47*(7), 850-853.

[4] Feder G et al. Guidelines for the prevention of falls in older people. BMJ, 2000, 321:1007-1011.

[5] Lord SR, Sherrington C, Menz HB. Falls in older people: risk factors and strategies for prevention. Cambridge University Press, 2000.

[6] https://www.aota.org/Conference-Events/OTMonth/what-is-OT.aspx. Accessed March 21, 2017

By addressing these extrinsic risk items, you will be able to eliminate 30%-50% of your risk of falling!

ACTION STEP

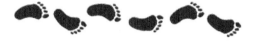

✓ Download and review the list of Extrinsic Risk Factors at Home from www.thebookofbalance.com/resources and repair or modify items that you have not checked off the list.

✓ Request your physician to review your medications with a strong risk association to falling.

CHAPTER 5

INTRINSIC RISK FACTORS

"Who looks outside, dreams; who looks inside, awakes."
- Carl Jung

While extrinsic risk factors for falls are mainly environmental causes that can easily be corrected or modified, intrinsic risk factors for falls often include medical conditions, diseases, and physical symptoms that are often intertwined and complex. It is highly recommended that these factors be thoroughly evaluated by your physical therapist or physician. Having a clear understanding of the interplay between the different intrinsic risk factors, and their effect on balance is paramount in improving your balance and decreasing your risk of falling.

In this chapter, we will examine the different intrinsic risk factors and how they can affect your balance.

SENSORY INPUTS for BALANCE

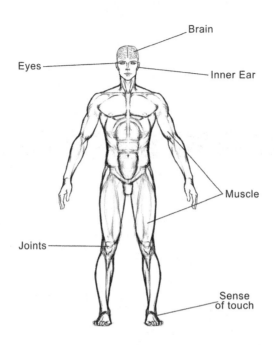

Balance Sensors

Posture and balance control results from a complex interplay between several sensory systems which involve perceiving environmental stimuli, responding to alterations in position, and maintaining your body's center of gravity within your base of support.[1]

It takes the three major sensory inputs: **vision**, **somatosensory**, and **vestibular system**, working together to give your brain the necessary information for your body to react appropriately to challenges to your posture or balance. To better understand how these three sensory inputs play a role in your balance, I will discuss each one in detail.

---

[1] Shaffer, S. W., and Harrison, A. L. (2007). Aging of the somatosensory system: a translational perspective. *Phys. Ther.* 87, 193–207. doi: 10.2522/ptj.20060083

1. Vision

As we get older, we become more and more visually dependent for our balance. I often witness this with my patients when I ask them to do the simple task of closing their eyes while standing. As soon as they close their eyes, their bodies start to sway, and they lose their equilibrium. Try it for yourself and see how long you can keep your body still while your eyes are closed.

contrast sensitivity ~ your ability to discern brightness or color that makes an object distinguishable.

If you cannot keep your balance with your eyes closed, it may mean that you have been relying a lot on your vision as your "balance compass."

Relying on your vision to keep your balance is not a huge problem in and of itself. In fact, your vision provides you with vital information about your environment and where you are in space. The problem of relying mainly on vision is aggravated when you develop vision impairments that come increasingly with age. These age-related changes in vision may include glaucoma, macular degeneration, cataract, astigmatism, and a myriad of other visual degenerative conditions. These various vision impairments, in varying degrees, affect your contrast sensitivity, depth perception, or ability to accommodate to low-light situations.

depth perception ~ your ability to perceive the relative distance of objects in your visual field.

These vision impairments, combined with an increasing reliance on vision for balance, can result to balance deficits and increased risk of falling.[2,3]

That explains part of the reason for Paul's recent falls. Paul has not seen his eye doctor for two years and has not had his prescription glasses updated for his latest vision needs. When he gets up in the morning and walks downstairs, his distorted depth perception affects his ability to gauge the height of the steps, literally causing him to take a "misstep."

As Paul makes his way to the poorly-lit hallway, his poor contrast sensitivity and difficulty to accommodate to low-light situations makes it hard for him to determine the distance and location of Martha's cats. Paul was not entirely exaggerating when he likened walking in a poorly-lit hallway filled with Martha's cats to that of navigating around landmines.

Another element of vision that is often overlooked is the *eye's tracking ability.* That is, are you able to follow moving objects with your gaze without getting dizzy or losing your balance?

The visual tracking ability is working in synchrony with the vestibular system to provide your brain with information to aid your balance whether your head is in motion, or when your head is still but your surrounding environment is in motion. When your visual and vestibular systems are not working together, a condition called *visual-vestibular mismatch* occurs. This condition can result in dizziness and imbalance.

A practical example of the visual system working together with the vestibular system in aiding your balance is when you are

---

[2] Freeman EE, Muñoz B, Rubin G, West SK. Visual field loss increases the risk of falls in older adults: the Salisbury Eye Evaluation. *Invest Ophthalmol Vis Sci.* 2007;48(10):4445-4450

[3] Lord SR. Visual risk factors for falls in older people. *Age Ageing.* 2006;35(suppl 2):ii42-ii45.

walking in crowded rooms. Trade and service areas, such as restaurants, supermarkets or shopping malls, airports, gas stations, or even public restrooms often have high-density traffic that bombards your senses with competing sensory inputs.

In these situations, you often need to be able to avoid collisions while filtering the "visual distractors" in the periphery.

I have patients tell me that they avoid going to supermarkets as much as they can. Looking at people milling around in different directions causes them to feel dizzy and lose their balance.

I also have patients telling me that they have totally stopped driving (which I highly recommend unless the problem is resolved) or even refrain from looking out of car windows for fear of getting dizzy.

Both scenarios are caused by the incongruent messages, or visual-vestibular mismatch, that the brain receives from the two sensory inputs. The movement of the surrounding environment that your eyes see does not correspond to the stillness of your head that the vestibular system perceives, or vice-versa.

The brain gets confused (or literally gets dizzy) from these diverging, often antagonizing messages. The result? A very high intrinsic risk of falling!

Fortunately, a simple set of multisensory exercises, done consistently, can often mitigate or resolve this problem by increasing the congruence of both visual and vestibular system functions. You will find these exercises in Part 2 of this book.

2. Somatosensory System

These are sensory inputs that come from your skin, muscles, and joints. These sensory inputs provide you with valuable information about muscle length and tension, joint movement and stress, touch, vibration, and pressure. They provide you with information about the position and movement of your body relative to the support surface beneath you.

The somatosensory system is involved in maintaining postural control and balance by making your body's muscular and skeletal frameworks aware of your body's spatial and mechanical status by providing you with a sense of your position and movement.

If you have an increased fear of falling, having maximum skin contact to a support surface while doing your exercises, i.e. sitting on a firm surface, will allow you to use the sensory inputs from a larger area of your body to inform you of your stability. My patients find it very reassuring that they can start their exercises to improve their balance in a sitting position.

As you get better in using the other systems (i.e. visual and vestibular) contributing to your balance, you will learn to maintain your balance even as you minimize your somatosensory inputs, i.e. exercising while standing on an unstable or compliant surface, or even standing on one leg. Just like your muscles, you are also able to improve the acuity of how you use your somatosensory system by performing exercises that pose a challenge to it.

3. Vestibular System

Your vision tells you about your position relative to your environment. Your somatosensory system provides you with information about your position relative to the support surface. What happens if you receive conflicting information from these two sensory systems? Who will be the judge? Who is the final arbiter?

That is the critical role of your vestibular system. The vestibular system identifies self-motion versus motion in the surrounding environment. It gathers information in how your head and body are positioned relative to gravity, speed, and direction. By filtering this information, your vestibular system helps you stabilize your posture and balance.

If your head is moving, your vestibular system stabilizes your visual gaze so you can focus on an object without getting dizzy or losing your balance. In contrast, if your head is still, it allows your gaze to follow moving objects in your environment without you getting dizzy.

Unfortunately, just as eye health and function decline with age, so does the vestibular system.

Two of the more common age-associated conditions seen with older adults are BPPV and Meniere's disease.

BPPV or *benign paroxysmal positional vertigo* is an inner ear condition that produces vertigo or attacks of a spinning sensation. *Benign* means a condition that is not injurious or malignant. *Paroxysmal* means a sudden or abrupt occurrence. *Positional* means that the condition results from a particular position or change in position. *Vertigo* is a dizzying sensation of tilting or spinning while you are within stable surroundings.

Described another way, whenever you change your position, more commonly when you tilt or turn your head, your surrounding environment starts to feel like its tilting or spinning, causing you to feel dizzy. Many of my patients liken the sensation to being seasick.

BPPV does not affect your hearing or vision. Instead, the issue emanates from the vestibular system found in your inner ear. In your inner ear are three fluid-filled canals called semicircular canals, each facing a different direction. Each time you turn or tilt your head, the fluid washes around the canals, bending the tiny hairs lined along the canals. Depending on the direction of where the tiny hairs bend, that is the information that is sent to your brain as to where your head is pointed.

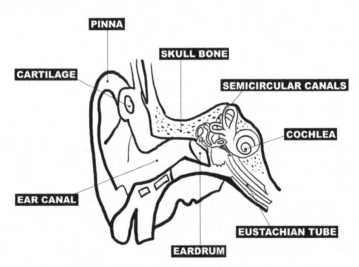

Inner Ear - Vestibular System

Moreover, there are tiny crystals stuck to these hairs whose function is to increase the sensitivity of the signals sent to your brain. With BPPV, these tiny crystals get loose, and they move around in your inner ear's semicircular canals. The movements of these loose crystals within the canals of your inner ear send incorrect signals to your brain.

When the vestibular system in your inner ear gives you different information from what your eyes are telling your brain, your brain gets confused. Or dizzy. Or BPPV.

This is what happened to my friend Betsy whom you met in the introduction of this book.

Several weeks before her fall, Betsy noticed that every time she would stoop down to put her shoes on, she would feel dizzy. The dizziness abated in less than a minute, so Betsy did not give much attention to it. What Betsy didn't know at that time was that each time she would stoop down, the displaced tiny crystals in her inner ear would float around the canals of her inner ear causing her to feel dizzy. The day she fell in her driveway, the position of stooping down to pick the newspaper from the ground triggered an attack of vertigo that caused her to lose her balance.

There are many other reasons and diagnoses, including central causes related to the brain and peripheral causes related to the inner ear, that can present with symptoms of dizziness or vertigo.

If you suspect that you have BPPV, I recommend that you see a physical therapist or physician specializing in vestibular rehabilitation. Your physical therapist or physician will perform a thorough assessment to eliminate other reasons for your dizziness, and they can also demonstrate and teach you the proper form and technique in performing corrective exercises.

tinnitus ~ a sensation of noise (such as ringing or roaring) which can only be heard by the one affected.

Meniere's disease can happen at any age, but it is more common in adults between 40 and 60 years of age. It is also a disorder of the inner ear that presents with symptoms of tinnitus, hearing loss, a feeling of fullness or congestion in the ear, and severe dizziness or vertigo.

otolaryngologist ~ doctor who specializes in the study and treatment of conditions of the ear, nose, and throat.

If you suspect that you have Meniere's disease, consult an otolaryngologist to have a proper diagnosis and treatment. Left untreated, some people experience "drop attacks," a sudden attack of severe vertigo that causes them to lose their balance and fall.

OTHER INTRINSIC FACTORS TO CONSIDER

Posture

Posture can change a person's center of gravity and impact their balance and functional ability. In 1947, the Posture Committee of the American Academy of Orthopedic Surgeons (AAOS) defined poor posture as a faulty relationship of the various parts of the body, which produce increased strain on the supporting structures, and in which there is a less efficient *balance* of the body over its base of support.

Imagine carrying a heavy bag on one side over a prolonged period. If you look from the front, the heavy load on one shoulder puts a postural strain on only one side of your body. Uneven postural strain, over time, fatigues and wears out the supporting structures of your body. Bones tend to reshape and adapt to the "new" postural demand. Muscles, being a contractile tissue, will either shorten or lengthen depending on which position the body is maintained over a prolonged period. Ligaments and cartilages tend to wear out sooner when uneven pressure or strain is applied over a prolonged period.

Have you noticed that one shoulder may be lower or higher than the other depending on which side a person is hand-dominant?

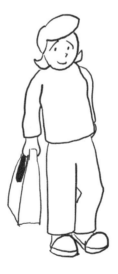

Uneven postural strain.

The same is true when you have poor posture as seen from the side. A lot of what you do every day is positioned in front of you. You lean or slouch forward when you eat, when you write, or whenever you work at a desk. People who work with computers often find themselves "sucked into" the computer. Once they get engrossed in what they are doing, you'll see their heads go forward toward the computer screen.

My patient Roberta has worked as an office secretary for over 30 years. She memorized the keys of a typewriter so that she could type up pages and pages of reports without looking at the keys of her typewriter. She told me how her tools of trade had evolved from using manual typewriters, the one where you would need to crank the lever on one side each time you finish typing one line, to using an electric typewriter, to eventually using a computer. She spent years slumped over her desk typing reports.

When I first saw Roberta, she was holding on to a walker with her head in a forward position and her shoulders rounded above the handles of her walker. You could almost visualize her still slumped forward into her typewriter or computer. No wonder her balance was off - her posture was off to begin with.

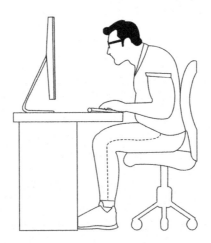

Forward head, rounded shoulder posture.

We all reach forward a lot more than we tend to reach back. This normal everyday function contributes to the tendency of the muscles in front of your body to be stronger than the muscles found in the back. If not countered with strengthening and postural exercises, the muscles, and the rest of the soft tissues on the front side of your body will shorten over time.

thoracic kyphosis ~ excessive hump position of the upper back.

These biomechanics often contribute to slouching while sitting or standing and causes your thoracic kyphosis to increase and your head and shoulders to slump forward. Not only does this position increase pressure on your internal organs, impeding breathing and circulation, it also shifts the line of gravity in your body, effectively changing your body's center of gravity.

The illustration below demonstrates the Plumb Line Test, a simple test you can do to see how your body aligns from the side and front. Another method would be to have somebody take your picture from the side and front or back views. As you look at your picture, put a ruler in the middle of your body and see if the ruler falls on the middle of your body or if your body is symmetrical from the front or back views.

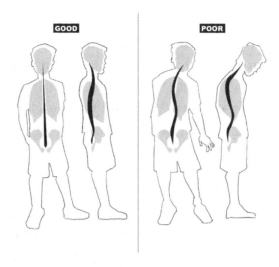

Plumb Line Test

Why is this important? Before progressing your strengthening exercises, it is critical to have your posture aligned appropriately. If you strengthen your muscles in a faulty posture, you will only be reinforcing the uneven strain that your poor posture applies to your body. Even if you get stronger from your exercise, your poor posture will result in an inefficient balance of your body.

Postural retraining that utilizes stretching, strengthening, and even biofeedback exercises are a great way to improve your posture and balance.

Before working on her balance, Roberta and I first worked on exercises to improve her posture. By *balancing the scale*, Roberta and I were able to improve her balance. After several weeks, she got rid of her walker. Roberta felt confident enough to walk without the aid of an assistive device!

Musculoskeletal

core muscles ~
group of muscles
that stabilize and
control your
abdomen, trunk,
and pelvis.

While leg-strengthening exercises are an important component of a balance program, and we will do a lot of leg-strengthening exercises in this book's program, an often-overlooked piece in a lot of balance programs is the role of the core muscles.

Think of your core muscles as the critical link in a chain connecting your upper and lower body. No matter how strong your upper or lower body is, if the core muscles that link them are weak, you will still end up with an unstable frame.

Remember our balance scale illustration in Chapter 1? Your core muscle is the pole in the middle of the scale. By supporting your spine, your core muscles can stabilize your body against challenges to your balance. Having a strong core will improve both your posture and balance. You will be addressing this very important component of your balance in Part 2 of this book.

Another often-overlooked component of a balance program is the role of flexibility and joint range of motion. Remember your ankle and hip strategies in Chapter 1? Your ankle and hip strategies help you maintain your balance by controlling how much your body sways to within your limits of stability. If your ankle or hip joints lack the flexibility to allow you to accommodate those body sways, your balance strategies are already compromised right from the get-go.

In Part 2 of this book, I will guide you through flexibility and strengthening exercises that will address your upper and lower body strength and flexibility.

CHAPTER 6

EXERCISE PHILOSOPHY AND SAFETY GUIDELINE

"Those who think they have no time to exercise will sooner or later have to find time for illness."
- Edward Stanley

I was fortunate to have met Linda early on in my career. She taught me an important lesson in patient care – if we, healthcare professionals, truly listen to our patients, they have just as much to teach us as we do to them. To quote Wendy Whelan, a retired principal dancer with the New York City Ballet, "We are constantly revealing ourselves to each other through our movement; learning from and teaching each other..."

Linda was a no-nonsense 73-year-old lady who grew up in the Midwest during the time of the Great Depression. She is a straight shooter who will tell you exactly what is in her mind, whether you like to hear it or not. When Linda was referred to me by her primary physician, she was hesitant to begin the balance program I designed for her. Linda lamented, "I understand the value of exercise but I've been to so many programs in my life, and I don't see how the exercises I've been doing are the *solutions* to my problems." Linda was looking for a solution to her balance problem, and she hadn't found it.

I asked Linda to elaborate on the different programs she had participated in and the specific exercises she has done so far. She proceeded to give me a dissertation on why the exercises did not make sense. Linda's honest answer taught me a valuable lesson that I have since incorporated into my clinical practice.

Exercise, for it to be effective, is not about being able to finish 10, 20, or 30 repetitions of leg lifts, squats, or heel and toe raises. Repetition alone, without usefulness or correlation to function, will not result in meaningful functional balance improvement.

Neither is exercise about being able to sit on a giant ball without falling. Linda doesn't want to be sitting on a giant ball while watching TV. She didn't need to be walking on a beam as if she was preparing for a tightrope exhibition either. These are great exercise ideas, but for Linda, it didn't translate to addressing her balance problems at home.

All Linda wanted to do was to be able to reach for a coffee mug from her cupboard without losing her balance, to step into her shower without feeling the need to grab onto the wall, or to walk out in her driveway without fear of the uneven terrain. She needed to be able to perform her daily activities in her own environment without fear of falling. All valid concerns.

functional training
~ exercises designed to develop dynamic strength, flexibility, coordination, and balance needed for everyday activities.

I designed this balance program based on two core exercise philosophies – first, the exercises should be based on functional training specific to the everyday tasks familiar to my patients. Second, the progression of the exercises should be based on each individual patient's fitness level and capabilities.

Specificity and Functional Task Integration

Professional swimmers sometimes perform yoga exercises to improve their flexibility, breathing, and relaxation techniques. This is called cross-training. Cross-training has the benefit of improving the performance of an athlete by adding to their skills a different skill set required to perform a different sport or activity.

Swimmers use cross-training to break the routine out of their own exercise program and have the added benefit of learning a different set of skills. But if a swimmer wants to hone his or her swimming skills, he or she will spend hours and hours in the pool every day repeating the same motion of their arms and legs over and over until muscle memory makes it an automatic response of their body.

That is the principle of specificity – if you want to learn to pitch a baseball, you need to practice pitching a baseball not practice shooting a basketball.

Why would it be different for you and your balance program?

Your balance exercise program should be task-specific. You don't need to jump up and down on a trampoline in your balance program if what challenges you every day is stepping up and down stairs. Every day, you are navigating challenges to your balance as you do your activities of daily living, e.g. getting up from a chair or toilet seat, stepping up or off a curb, walking with a glass of water in one hand, or walking while talking on your phone. Your exercise program should be designed around those challenges. It should integrate the common functional tasks you do every day. The best way to relearn a given task is to train specifically for that task.[1]

The exercises in this program are designed to assist you in activities that you will most likely be doing at home or in your community. If you need help in getting up from a chair, spend more time training and practicing getting up from a chair. If you feel unsteady using the stairs or stepping up or off a curb, train and practice those tasks. Be specific to your individual needs, and integrate your daily function into the exercise movements in this program.

By practicing the different balance reactions and strategies you will learn from this book, your body will know how to react to any given situation because your brain and body have rehearsed it over and over.

Principle of Exercise Progression

More than twenty years of being a physical therapist have taught me that if the exercises are too easy for a patient and they do not feel challenged, they will soon lose interest and stop doing their exercises. On the other hand, if the exercises

---

[1] Bayona NA, Bitensky J, Salter K, Teasell R. The role of task-specific training in rehabilitation therapies. Top Stroke Rehabil. 2005 Summer;12(3):58-65

are too difficult to perform and patients keep on failing, they are more likely to give up.

As clinicians, we sometimes assume, often mistakenly, that patients are being non-compliant if they do not do the exercises we prescribe. Once we spend the time to ask and really listen to our patients, the reason they cite fall into either one of the two answers above.

I designed this program to meet you at the level of confidence, skill, capability, and fitness you are in. There is a gradual increase in the volume, intensity, or complexity of the exercises. You will not be walking on a balance beam if you cannot hold your balance while standing still on solid ground!

The exercises you will be doing from one level to the next are designed to prepare your body for the increasing challenges required to be successful at the next level. The program starts from the easiest to perform, progressing to the more difficult or complex.

Though the first few levels would look too easy to some, to get the best result, I highly recommend that you go through the exercise level progression from the very first level before going on to the next. Spend time at each level until you feel comfortable enough to proceed to the next.

In the same token, if you have difficulty mastering any one level, do not give up. Keep at it until you improve your balance enough for your body to be ready for the next level of exercises. Just like an athlete in training – the more times you do it, the better you'll be at it. The better you are in performing the exercises, the better your balance will be.

Exercise Safety Guideline

Before starting the exercise program, I highly recommend that you first consult your physical therapist or physician if you have any physical or medical condition that may put you at risk of injury. Always exercise according to your fitness level and capability. Start slow and focus on proper body alignment until you can execute the movements using proper form.

Warm-up. Warm-ups prepare your body's physiological response to exercise by redistributing blood flow from your internal organs to the muscles that you will be exercising. By doing warm-up exercises, you are reducing your risk of injuries. A good warm-up exercise typically consists of 5-10 minutes of low to moderate intensity walking, stationary bike, or marching in seating or standing positions.

Watch your form and posture. Keep your back aligned with a neutral spine. Engage your stomach muscles.

Don't bounce your stretch. Ballistic stretching (bouncing while stretching) can increase the chance of muscle tears. Gentle sustained stretch held for at least 30 seconds is an effective way to improve your flexibility.

"No pain, no gain" is not true. Exercise should require some effort and be a little uncomfortable; however, pain of the sharp, acute, or recurring kind, is a warning sign you should not ignore. If you have rheumatoid arthritis, osteoarthritis, back or neck pain, or other painful conditions, perform your exercises in a pain-free range. Consult your physical therapist or physician if you have continuing pain during exercise.

Breathe. Never hold your breath. Proper breathing techniques are essential when training.

Eyes open before eyes closed. Do not progress to exercises with your eyes closed if you are not able to perform the exercise safely with your eyes open.

Stop. Stop performing any exercise if you experience chest pain, dizziness, shortness of breath, or if you get disoriented.

Do not proceed. Do not progress to the next level until the prior level is performed successfully without imbalance.

Cool-down. The cool-down is the first step in the recovery process. Your body's ability to recover from exercise is impeded when you neglect the cool-down phase. A good cool-down exercise typically consists of 5-10 minutes of low-intensity walking, stationary bike, or stretching.

PART 2

LEVEL 1

BIOMECHANICAL EXERCISES
(To improve posture, flexibility, and strength.)

1. Static Back Stretch

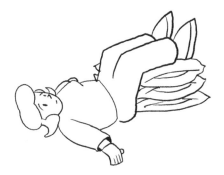

a. Lie on your back with your legs propped up on pillows so that your hips and knees are at a 90-degree angle.
b. Put your arms as close as possible to the level of your shoulders.
c. Stay in this position for 3-5 minutes or until your neck and back relaxes and settles into proper alignment.

Why? This will relax your back and position your head in the same plane as your shoulders – a great antidote to a forward head, rounded shoulder position you are stuck with for most of the day. Not only is this exercise easy to do, your neck and back will feel great too!

2. Supine Frog Stretch

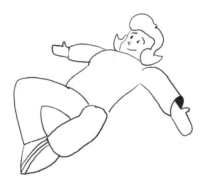

a. Lie on your back with your feet together and your knees apart.
b. With your palms facing up, place your arms as close to shoulder level as possible.
c. Relax in this position for 2 minutes, then return to your original position.
d. Repeat the exercise 3-5 times.

Why? The frog position will loosen the muscles in your groin, inner thighs, and back, giving you more flexibility to perform your hip strategy for balance.

3. Supine Lumbar Rotation

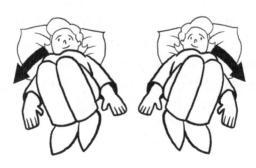

a. Lie on your back with your feet and knees together.
b. Bend both knees, so your feet are flat on the bed or floor.
c. Slowly rotate your back, so your knees move from side-to-side.
d. Repeat the exercise 10 times.

Why? This exercise will help loosen up your back and hips giving you more flexibility to perform your hip and stepping strategies for balance.

4. Supine Hip Flexor Stretch

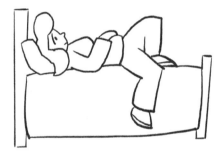

a. Scoot to the side of the bed so that you can slowly lower one leg off the edge of the bed.
b. To help support your back, bend the knee of the leg that stays on the bed.
c. Hold this position for 1 minute and repeat 5 times.
d. Scoot on the other side of the bed and perform the same exercise for the other leg.

Why? Prolonged sitting during the day shorten the muscles in front of your hips and groin, causing you to lean forward on your hips once you stand up and walk. Having tight or shortened muscles in front of your hips will cause you to lean forward; affecting your posture and balance while standing.

5. Supine Hamstring Stretch

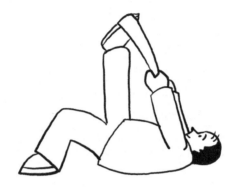

a. Lie on your back and raise one knee up using a towel or belt wrapped around your foot.
b. Keep the knee of the leg you are raising as straight as you can.
c. Hold the stretch for 1 minute and return to your original position.
d. Repeat 5 times for each leg.

Why? In the same manner that prolonged sitting shortens the muscles in front of your hips, it also shortens the muscles at the back of your thighs. To compensate for tight hamstring muscles, a lot of people lean forward while slightly bending their knees to "balance" their body. Over time, tight hamstring muscles contribute to the "slouched standing" posture.

6. Seated Calf Stretch

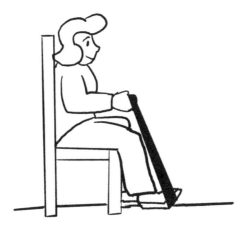

a. Sit erect with both feet flat on the floor.
b. Loop a towel or belt around the ball of one foot just below your toes.
c. Keep your heel on the floor while gently pulling the towel, allowing your foot to bend up to your knee.
d. Hold the stretch for 1 minute and return to your original position.
e. Repeat 5 times for each leg.

Why? Stretching your ankle in this position targets the muscles behind your leg. Keeping your calf muscles flexible will allow you to react quicker using your ankle strategy to maintain your balance.

7. Seated Push-up

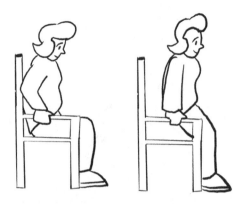

a. Sit erect on a chair with both feet flat on the floor.
b. Place your hands on the armrests of the chair and press down, raising your buttocks off the chair.
c. Extend your arms straight to lift your buttocks off the chair.
d. Slowly bend your elbows to lower your buttocks back to the chair.
e. Perform 10 repetitions for 2-3 sets.

Why? This exercise will strengthen the muscles of your upper back, shoulders, and arms to aid getting up from a chair.

8. Seated Leg Extension

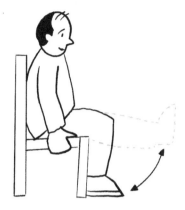

a. Sit erect on a chair with both feet flat on the floor.
b. Extend one leg until it is parallel to the floor.
c. Hold the position for 2-3 seconds before slowly lowering the leg on the floor.
d. Perform 10 repetitions for 2-3 sets on each side.

Why? This exercise will strengthen the muscles in the front of your thighs. This muscle not only helps extend your knee when you get up from a sitting position, it is also crucial in keeping your balance when you are standing still or walking.

9. Seated Hip Flexion

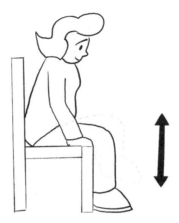

a. Sit erect on a chair with both feet flat on the floor.
b. Lift one foot up off the floor by raising your knee as high as you can.
c. Hold the position for 2-3 seconds before lowering your foot back to the floor.
d. Perform 10 repetitions for 2-3 sets on each side.

Why? This exercise will strengthen the muscles in your groin and the front of your hips. In addition to their major function of bending your hips during your hip and stepping strategies for balance, their attachment to your spine makes them an important part of your core muscles to help stabilize your spine.

10. Seated Heel/Toe Raises

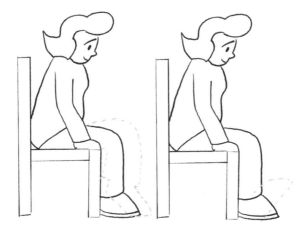

a. Sit erect on a chair with both feet flat on the floor.
b. Raise your toes as high as you can while keeping your heels on the ground.
c. Bring your toes down back to original position.
d. Raise your heels as high as you can while keeping your toes on the ground.
e. Bring your heels down back to their original position.
f. Perform 15 repetitions for 2-3 sets.

Why? This is a great exercise to improve your ankle flexibility and strength. This will come in handy as you work on your ankle strategies in the higher levels of your balance program.

STABILIZATION EXERCISES
(To improve trunk and posture control.)

1. Supported Front/Back Weight Shifting

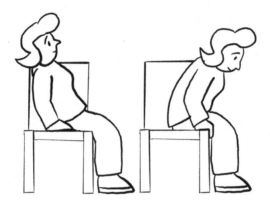

a. Sit erect with both feet flat on the floor, hands on your lap or chair for support.

b. Lean forward through your hips, bringing your nose over your knees.

c. Hold the position for 3-5 seconds then return to the starting position.

d. Lean backward through your hips.

e. Hold the position for 3-5 seconds then return to the starting position.

f. Perform 10 repetitions in each direction.

Why? Having strong stomach and trunk muscles will improve your ability to control your posture and balance when you lean backward or reach forward.

2. Supported Side-to-Side Weight Shifting

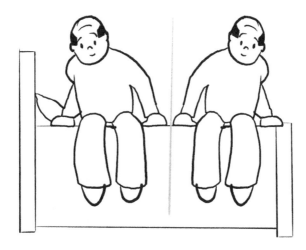

a. Sit erect with both feet flat on the floor, hands holding on the chair for support.

b. Lean your head, shoulder, and arm so that your weight is shifted toward one side.

c. Hold the position for 3-5 seconds then return to the starting position.

d. Lean toward the opposite side.

e. Hold the position for 3-5 seconds then return to the starting position.

f. Perform 10 repetitions in each direction.

Why? This exercise will help with your ability to control your posture and balance when you perform functional activities requiring you to bend or reach in multiple directions.

3. Segmental Neck and Trunk Rotation

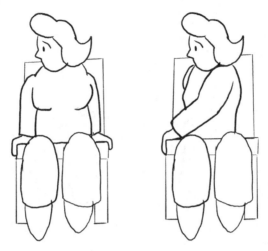

a. Sit erect with both feet flat on the floor.
b. With your knees together, first rotate your neck to one side, followed by your trunk rotating toward the same side.
c. Hold the position for 3-5 seconds.
d. Return to the starting position then perform on the other side.
e. Perform 10 repetitions in each direction.

Why? This exercise will improve your ability to look over your shoulder without losing your balance.

MULTISENSORY TRAINING
(To optimize use and function of sensory systems.)

1. Side-to-Side Head Motion, Eyes Open

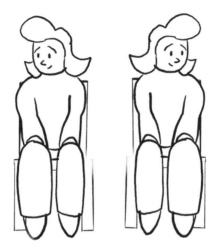

a. Sit erect with both feet flat on the floor, hands resting on your lap or chair.

b. Move your head from one side to the other at a speed you are comfortable with.

c. Keep your eyes open as you focus on objects from side-to-side.

d. Repeat 10 times.

Why? This exercise will improve your ability to control your eye movements as you move your head from side-to-side, reducing episodes of dizziness or loss of balance when you look or move your head from side-to-side.

2. Up and Down Head Motion, Eyes Open

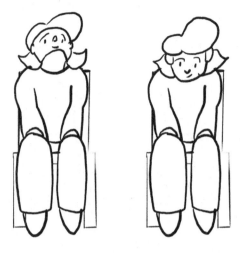

a. Sit erect with both feet flat on the floor, hands resting on your lap or chair.
b. Move your head to look up and down at a speed you are comfortable with.
c. Keep your eyes open as you focus on objects from the floor to the ceiling.
d. Repeat 10 times.

Why? This exercise will improve your ability to control your eye movements as you move your head up and down, reducing episodes of dizziness or loss of balance when you look or move your head up and down.

3. Side-to-Side Head Motion, Eyes Closed

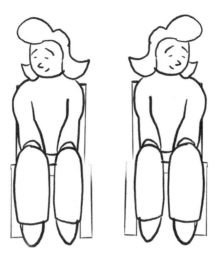

a. Sit erect with both feet flat on the floor, hands resting on your lap or chair.

b. With your eyes closed, move your head from one side to the other at a speed you are comfortable with.

c. Repeat 10 times.

Why? By eliminating your visual feedback, you sharpen your sense of touch and inner ear systems to help keep your balance when you move your head or look side-to-side in a low-light situation.

4. Up and Down Motion, Eyes Closed

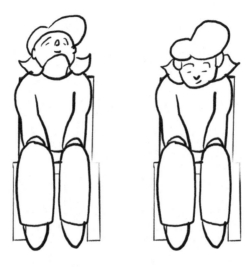

a. Sit erect with both feet flat on the floor, hands resting on your lap or chair.
b. With your eyes closed, move your head up and down at a speed you are comfortable with.
c. Repeat 10 times.

Why? By eliminating your visual feedback, you sharpen your sense of touch and inner ear systems to help keep your balance when you move your head or look up and down in a low-light situation.

STEP TRAINING
(To improve agility, coordination, and reaction time.)

1. Half-star Stepping in Sitting Position

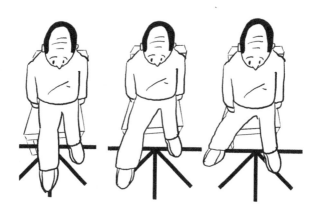

a. Sit erect with both feet flat on the floor.

b. Set your metronome to between 30-60 beats per minute (bpm), depending on your comfort level and reaction time.

c. Follow each beat of the metronome by stepping as far as you can to each point of an imaginary half-star on the floor.

d. Perform 2-3 sets of 2 minutes.

Tip #1: If you do not have a metronome, you can use a free metronome by searching "metronome" on Google, or you can download a free app on your smartphone.

Tip #2: Start with the lowest number of beats per minute you are comfortable with, and as your reaction time improves, increase the frequency of the metronome by 5-10 bpm until you reach 60 bpm or higher.

Why? This exercise will improve your stepping strategy by improving your reaction time and increasing the accuracy of your foot placement.

LEVEL 2

BIOMECHANICAL EXERCISES
(To improve posture, flexibility, and strength.)

1. Turtle Neck

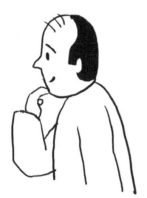 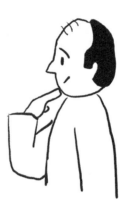

a. Sit erect with both feet flat on the floor.
b. While keeping your eyes focused on an object in front of you, place your fingertips on your chin.
c. Gently tuck in your chin, then draw your head back toward your shoulders.
d. Return to the starting position.
e. Perform 10-15 repetitions.

Why? This exercise will not only help correct the "forward head posture," it is also effective at treating chronic neck pain that is caused by the daily stresses of poor posture while sitting or standing.

2. Side Neck Stretch

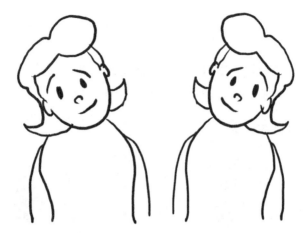

a. Sit erect with both feet flat on the floor.
b. Tilt your head toward one side until you feel a stretch on the muscles on the opposite side of your neck.
c. Hold for 15 seconds.
d. Return to the starting position.
e. Perform 10 repetitions on each side.

Why? This exercise will improve the flexibility of your neck, it is especially important if you tend to keep your head in one position for long periods of time, i.e. reading or watching TV.

3. Butterfly Stretch

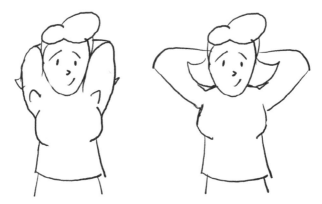

a. Sit erect with both feet flat on the floor.
b. While raising both elbows in front of you, reach for your ears with your hands on both sides.
c. Keeping your hands on your ears, open your elbows out to the side as far as you can until you feel a stretch in front of your chest.
d. Hold the position for 30 seconds.
e. Slowly return to the starting position.
f. Perform 5-8 repetitions.

Why? This exercise will stretch the muscles in front of your chest that tend to tighten as you spend hours during the day sitting or slumped in a "rounded shoulders" position.

4. Seated Spine and Arm Extension

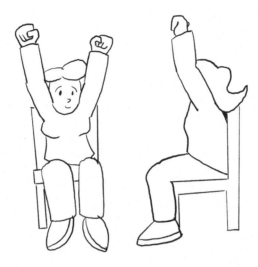

a. Sit erect with both feet flat on the floor.
b. Raise both arms up in front of you.
c. Reach as high as you can while extending your spine.
d. Hold for 3-5 seconds.
e. Slowly return to the starting position.
f. Perform 5-8 repetitions.

Why? This exercise will help straighten your spine and improve your posture - a great antidote to a "slumped posture."

5. Shoulder Elevation

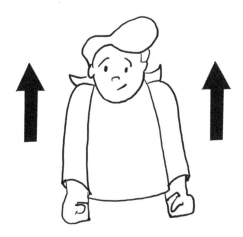

a. Sit erect with both feet flat on the floor.
b. Bring both shoulders up as high as you can.
c. Hold the position for 3-5 seconds.
d. Slowly lower both shoulders back to the starting position.
e. Perform 8-10 repetitions.

Why? This exercise will strengthen the muscles of your upper back and shoulders to help correct the "forward head, rounded shoulders" posture.

6. Shoulder Retraction

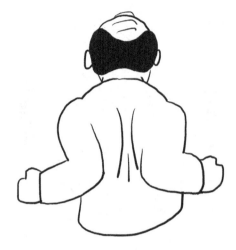

    a. Sit erect with both feet flat on the floor.
    b. Squeeze both shoulder blades together by pressing your elbows toward your spine.
    c. Hold the position for 3-5 seconds.
    d. Slowly return to the starting position.
    e. Perform 8-10 repetitions.

Why? This exercise will strengthen the muscles in between your shoulder blades, helping correct the "rounded shoulders" posture.

7. Round to Straight Back

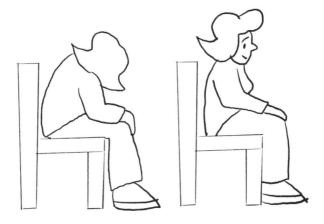

a. Sit erect with both feet flat on the floor.
b. Relax your back muscles and round your back by slumping your trunk forward.
c. Slowly extend your spine by tightening your back and abdominal muscles.
d. Perform 8-10 repetitions.

Why? This exercise will improve your awareness of the position of your back and increase your control of your back and stomach muscles. This is also a great exercise to align your back and relieve pain and stiffness while reading or watching TV.

8. Seated Elbow to Knee Abdominal Strengthening

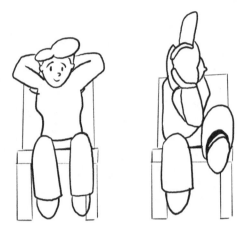

a. Sit erect with both feet flat on the floor.
b. Place your hands on the side of your head in a butterfly position.
c. Lift one knee to reach the opposite elbow by slowly twisting your trunk.
d. Slowly return to the starting position.
e. Perform 2 sets of 15 repetitions.

Why? This exercise will strengthen your core and the muscles at the sides of your stomach. Having strong muscles at the sides of your stomach will stabilize your trunk and keep your balance when you turn around or reach for objects with your opposite hand.

9. Seated Abdominal Crunches

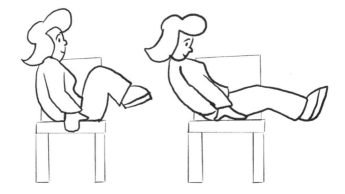

a. Sit on a sturdy chair and hold onto the sides of the chair for support.
b. Ease back slightly, and draw both knees up.
c. Perform crunches by extending your legs out and bringing your legs in toward your chest while contracting your abs.
d. Perform 2 sets of 15 repetitions.

Why? This exercise will strengthen your core muscles. Your core muscles act as the corset of your body, stabilizing your entire body to give you better balance when you move around.

STABILITY EXERCISES
(To improve trunk and posture control.)

1. Unsupported Front/Back Weight Shifting

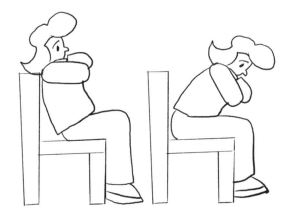

a. Sit erect with both feet flat on the floor, arms crossed on your chest.
b. Lean forward through your hips, bringing your nose over your knees.
c. Hold the position for 3-5 seconds, then return to the starting position.
d. Lean backward through hips.
e. Hold the position for 3-5 seconds, then return to the starting position.
f. Perform 10 repetitions in each direction.

Why? This is a progression of the supported front/back weight-shifting exercise you performed in Level 1. This exercise will improve your ability to control your posture and balance when you lean forward or backward without using your hands for support.

2. Unsupported Side-to-Side Weight Shift

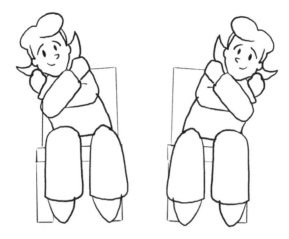

a. Sit erect with both feet flat on the floor, arms crossed on your chest.

b. Lean your body toward one side as far as you can without losing your balance.

c. Hold the position for 3-5 seconds, then return to the starting position.

d. Lean toward the opposite side.

e. Hold the position for 3-5 seconds, then return to the starting position.

f. Perform 10 repetitions in each direction.

Why? This is a progression of the side-to-side weight-shifting exercise you performed in Level 1. This exercise will improve your ability to control your posture and balance when you reach for objects on your side.

3. Sitting Twist and Turn

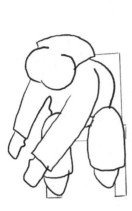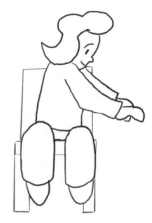

a. Sit erect with both feet flat on the floor.
b. Imagine picking up objects on the right side of the floor and placing it up on your left side.
c. Return to the original position.
d. Imagine picking up objects on the left side of the floor and placing it up on your right side.
e. Return to the original position.
f. Perform 10 repetitions on each side.

Why? This exercise will increase the strength of your core and trunk muscles to improve your trunk control and balance during functional activities requiring trunk rotation.

MULTISENSORY TRAINING
(To optimize use and function of sensory systems.)

1. Forward Arm Raises, Eyes Closed

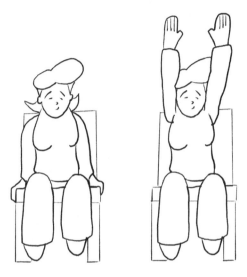

a. Sit erect with both feet flat on the floor.
b. With your eyes closed, raise both arms up in front of you.
c. Hold position for 3-5 seconds.
d. Slowly return to the starting position, then open your eyes.
e. Perform 8-10 repetitions for 2 sets.

Why? By eliminating your visual feedback, you sharpen your sense of touch and inner ear systems to help keep your balance during low-light situations.

2. Side Arm Raises, Eyes Closed

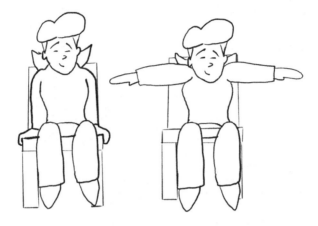

a. Sit erect with both feet flat on the floor.
b. With your eyes closed, raise both arms up in your side.
c. Hold the position for 3-5 seconds.
d. Slowly return to the starting position, then open your eyes.
e. Perform 8-10 repetitions for 2 sets.

Why? By eliminating your visual feedback, you sharpen your sense of touch and inner ear systems to help keep your balance during low-light situations.

3. Smooth Pursuit in Sitting

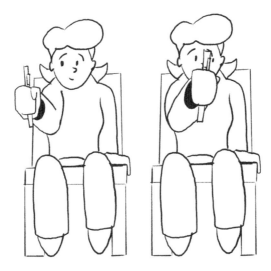

a. Sit erect with both feet flat on the floor.
b. Hold a pen (or business card) in front of you.
c. Keep your head still while your eyes are focused on the pen.
d. Move the pen (or business card) from side-to-side or up/down, following it with your eyes only.
e. Perform 15-20 repetitions for 2-3 sets.

Tip: Start this exercise with slow movement and gradually increase to a more rapid rate as your tolerance and level of comfort improves.

Why? This exercise will re-train the movement of your eyes, independently of your head. The goal of this exercise is for your brain to learn to tolerate and accurately interpret information coming from your different sensory systems.

4. Saccades in Sitting

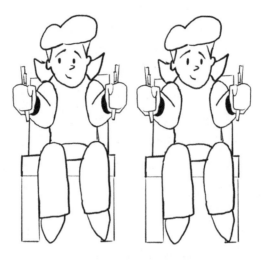

a. Sit erect with both feet flat on the floor.
b. Hold two pens (or business cards) placed about 12 inches apart in front of you.
c. Keep your head still, and move your eyes quickly to focus on the pens from side-to-side.
d. Perform 15-20 repetitions for 2-3 sets.

Why? This exercise will re-train the movement of your eyes, independently of your head. As your brain learns to adapt to these eye movements, you will find that your tolerance to look quickly in different directions without getting dizzy will improve. This skill comes in handy when you are walking in crowded areas or when you must look quickly at different targets without losing your balance.

5. Gaze Stabilization in Sitting

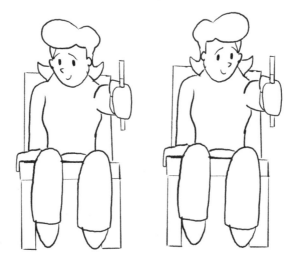

a. Sit erect with both feet flat on the floor.
b. Hold a pen (or business card) in front of you.
c. Keep your eyes focused on the pen while moving your head from side-to-side or up/down.
d. Perform 15-20 repetitions for 2-3 sets.

Tip: The pen (or business card) must remain in focus, not blurry, and appear stationary while your head is in motion. Start this exercise with slow movement and gradually increase to a more rapid rate as long as the target remains in focus.

Why? This exercise will help stabilize your focus independently of your head movement. As your brain learns to adapt to these head movements, you will find that you can maintain your focus on a target even when you are moving your head. This skill comes in handy when you need to focus on a stationary target even as your head or body is moving; for instance, while walking in a crowded street.

STEP TRAINING
(To improve agility, coordination, and reaction time.)

1. Stepping Exercise in Sitting + Cognitive Task

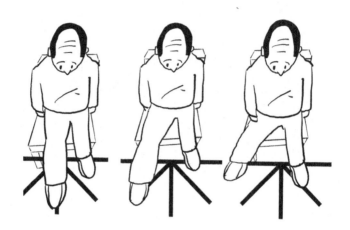

a. Sit erect with both feet flat on the floor.

b. Set your metronome to between 30-60 beats per minute (bpm), depending on your comfort level and reaction time.

c. Follow each beat of the metronome by stepping as far as you can to each point of an imaginary half-star on the floor.

d. Perform this stepping exercise while you have your TV on in front of you. This will add another task demanding your attention while you perform your stepping exercise.

e. Repeat 2-3 sets of 2 minutes each.

Tip: Start with the lowest number of beats per minute you are comfortable with, and as your reaction time improves, increase the frequency of the metronome by 5-10 bpm until you reach 60 bpm.

Why? This is a dual-task exercise that will improve your stepping strategy for balance while performing two different tasks simultaneously.

LEVEL 3

BIOMECHANICAL EXERCISES
(To improve posture, flexibility, and strength.)

1. Door Stretch

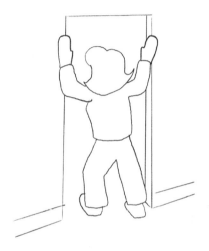

    a. Stand in a doorframe and place your arms out to your sides, placing your forearms against the frame.

    b. Slowly lean or step forward until you feel a light stretch in the chest and shoulders.

    c. Hold this stretch for 30 seconds, and return to the starting position.

    d. Perform 8-10 repetitions.

Why? This exercise will improve your posture by stretching the tight muscles in your chest and shoulders.

2. "W" Wall Stretch

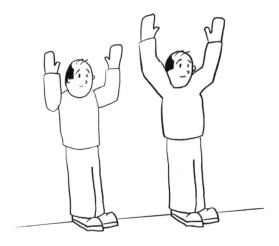

   a. Stand with your upper back and buttocks against a wall.

   b. Raise both arms to the side with the back of your hands against the wall.

   c. Slowly slide both hands up as high as you can, keeping the back of your hands and elbows against the wall.

   d. Slowly slide both hands down to get back to their original position.

   e. Perform 8-10 repetitions.

Why? This exercise will improve your posture by aligning your head and spine in one plane while stretching your arm and shoulder muscles.

3. Standing Hip Abductor Stretch

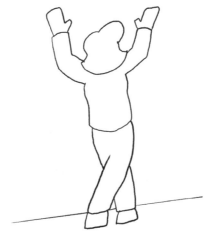

a. Stand 8-12 inches from a wall and place both hands on the wall for support.

b. Cross your right leg behind your left leg.

c. While maintaining both feet on the floor, push your right hip to the side until you feel a stretch.

d. Hold the stretch for 30 seconds, then return to the original position.

e. Perform 5 repetitions on each side.

Why? This exercise will improve the flexibility of the muscles on the side of your hips, making your hip and stepping strategies easier to perform.

4. Standing Hip Flexor Stretch

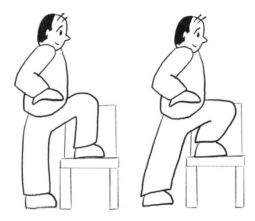

a. Stand 8-12 inches from a chair and place your left foot on the seat of a chair.

b. While keeping your trunk upright, bring your left knee forward until you feel a stretch on your right hip.

c. Hold the stretch for 30 seconds, then return to the original position.

d. Repeat instructions on the other leg.

e. Perform 5 repetitions on each side.

Why? This exercise will improve the flexibility of the muscles in front of your hips, making your hip and stepping strategies easier to perform.

5. Standing Calf Stretch

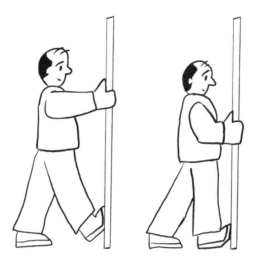

a. Stand 8-12 inches away from a wall.

b. Tilt one foot up against the wall while keeping the heel down on the floor.

c. Lean your body forward until you feel a stretch at the back of your leg.

d. Hold the stretch for 30 seconds, then return to the original position.

e. Perform 8-10 repetitions on each side.

Why? This exercise will improve the flexibility of the muscles in your leg and foot, making your ankle strategy easier to perform.

STABILITY EXERCISES
(To improve trunk and posture control.)

1. Standing Forward Reach

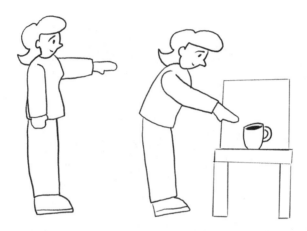

    a. Stand 15 inches away from an object placed in front of you.

    b. Without moving your feet, reach as far forward as you can toward the object without losing your balance.

    c. Return to the original position.

    d. Perform 8-10 repetitions with each hand.

Why? This exercise will increase your "margin of stability" by improving your ability to control your trunk and posture. Improving your trunk and posture control will help you maintain your balance while performing functional activities.

2. Standing Side Reach

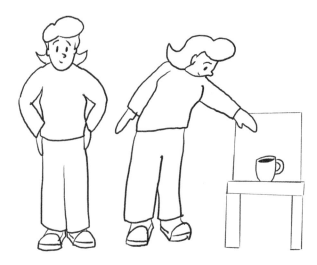

a. Stand 15 inches away from an object placed at your side.

b. Without moving your feet, reach as far as you can toward the object at your side without losing your balance.

c. Return to the original position.

d. Perform 8-10 repetitions on each side.

Why? This exercise will increase your "margin of stability" by improving your ability to control your trunk and posture. Improving your trunk and posture control will help you maintain your balance while reaching for objects on your side.

3. Forward/Backward Weight Shift

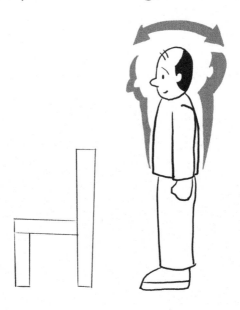

a. Stand near a counter or chair to hold onto in case of balance loss.

b. Leading with your upper body, gently lean forward until you feel your body weight shift toward the ball of your feet or your toes.

c. Return to the original position.

d. Leading with your upper body, gently lean backward until you feel your body weight shift toward the heels of your feet.

e. Return to the original position.

f. Perform 8-10 repetitions in each direction.

Why? This exercise will improve your ankle strategy by strengthening your postural muscles. This will also increase your awareness of your center of gravity and the limits of your stability.

4. Side-to-Side Weight Shift

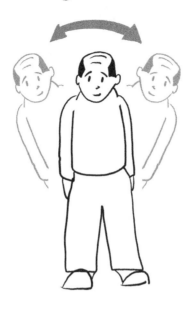

a. Stand near a counter or chair to hold onto in case of balance loss.

b. Leading with your upper body, gently lean toward your right side until you feel your body weight shift toward your right foot.

c. Return to the original position.

d. Leading with your upper body, gently lean toward your left side until you feel your body weight shift toward your left foot.

e. Return to the original position.

f. Perform 8-10 repetitions in each direction.

Why? This exercise will strengthen your postural muscles as well as increase your awareness of your center of gravity and the limits of your stability.

TRANSITION EXERCISES
(To prevent balance loss when changing positions.)

1. Sit to Stand

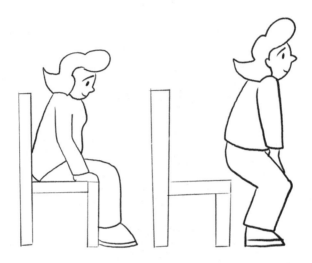

 a. Sit erect with your feet hip-width apart on the floor.

 b. Slide your buttocks closer to the front of the chair so that the front of your knees are in line with your toes.

 c. While keeping your back straight, lean your upper body forward.

 d. Push your feet down and extend your hips to get into a standing position.

 e. Slowly sit back into the chair, keeping the muscles in front of your thighs engaged until your buttocks rest on the chair.

 f. Perform 8-10 repetitions.

Tip: You can start by pushing up on the armrests of the chair to help you get into a standing position. As you get stronger, perform the exercise without using your hands.

Why? Sit to stand is a great functional exercise to strengthen the muscles in your thighs and buttocks.

2. Alternating Touch Step

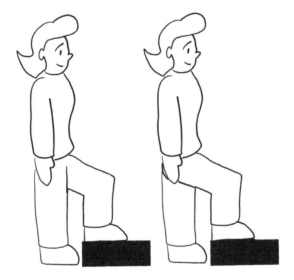

a. Stand 6-8 inches in front of a box or step stool.
b. Alternately place your left and right foot on the box or step stool as if you are marching in place.
c. Perform 15 steps on each side.

Why? This exercise will improve your ability to shift your weight from one foot to the other without losing your balance.

3. Standing Heel/Toe Raises

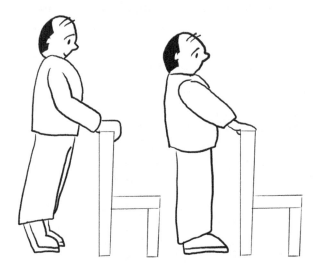

a. Stand in front of a chair or counter.
b. While holding on to the chair or counter, alternately raise your heels and toes up as high as you can.
c. Perform 25-30 repetitions.

Why? This exercise will strengthen the muscles of your legs and feet while increasing your awareness of the limits of your stability.

MULTISENSORY TRAINING
(To optimize use and function of sensory systems.)

1. Standing Forward Arm Raises with Eyes Closed

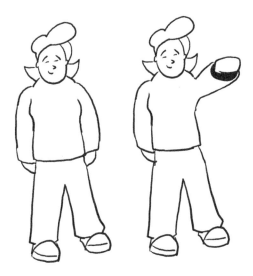

a. Stand with your feet hip-width apart.
b. With your eyes closed, alternately raise your left and right arms up in front of you.
c. Perform 3 sets of 10 repetitions each.

Why? By eliminating your visual feedback, you sharpen your inner ear function and your sense of touch on the soles of your feet.

2. Standing Side Arm Raises with Eyes Closed

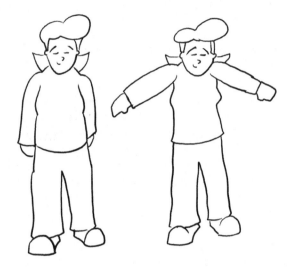

    a. Stand with your feet hip-width apart.
    b. With your eyes closed, raise both left and right arms up on your side.
    c. Perform 3 sets of 10 repetitions each.

Why? By eliminating your visual feedback, you sharpen your inner ear function and your sense of touch on the soles of your feet.

3. Standing Smooth Pursuit

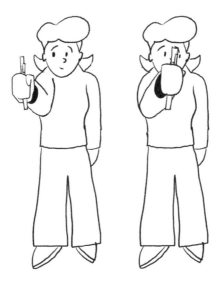

a. Stand with your feet hip-width apart.
b. Hold a pen (or business card) in front of you.
c. Keep your head still while your eyes are focused on the pen.
d. Move the pen (or business card) from side-to-side or up/down, following it with your eyes only.
e. Perform 15-20 repetitions for 2-3 sets.

Tip: Start this exercise with slow movement and gradually increase to a more rapid rate as your tolerance and level of comfort improves.

Why? This exercise is a progression of the smooth pursuit exercise you did while sitting. By standing, you are reducing your surface support and feedback from the wider surface of your buttocks when you are sitting, to a smaller surface support, the soles of your feet when you are standing.

4. Standing Saccade

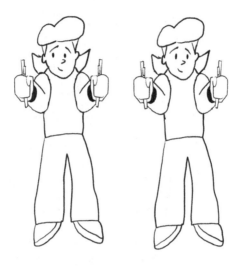

a. Stand with your feet hip-width apart.
b. Hold two pens (or business cards) placed about 12 inches apart in front of you.
c. Keep your head still and move your eyes quickly to focus on the pens (or business cards) from side-to-side or up/down.
d. Perform 15-20 repetitions for 2-3 sets.

Why? This exercise is a progression of the saccade exercise you did while sitting. By standing, you are reducing your surface support and feedback from the wider surface of your buttocks when you are sitting, to a smaller surface support, the soles of your feet when you are standing.

5. Standing Gaze Stabilization

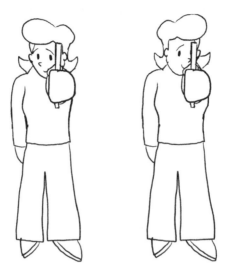

a. Sit erect with both feet flat on the floor.
b. Hold a pen (or business card) in front of you.
c. Keep your eyes focused on the pen while moving your head from side-to-side or up and down.
d. Perform 15-20 repetitions for 2-3 sets.

Tip: The pen (or business card) must remain in focus, not blurry, and appear stationary while your head is in motion. Start this exercise with slow movement and gradually increase to a more rapid rate as long as the target remains in focus.

Why? This exercise is a progression of the gaze stabilization exercise you did while sitting. By standing, you are reducing your surface support and feedback from the wider surface of your buttocks when you are sitting, to a smaller surface support, the soles of your feet when you are standing.

STEP TRAINING
(To improve agility, coordination, and reaction time.)

1. Star Stepping

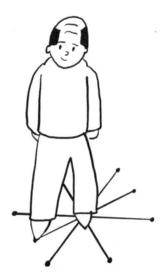

a. Stand in the middle of an imaginary star on the floor.

b. Set your metronome to between 30-60 beats per minute (bpm), depending on your comfort level and reaction time.

c. Follow each beat of the metronome by stepping as far as you can to each point of an imaginary star on the floor.

d. Repeat 2-3 sets of 2 minutes each.

Tip #1: Start with the lowest number of beats per minute you are comfortable with, and as your reaction time improves, increase the frequency of the metronome by 5-10 bpm until you reach 60 bpm.

Tip #2: Take a large step, because only with a large step can you effectively catch yourself if you lose your balance.

Why? This is a progression of the step training you performed while sitting. This exercise will improve your stepping strategy by increasing the accuracy of your foot placement, and improving your reaction time and coordination.

LEVEL 4

BIOMECHANICAL EXERCISES
(To improve posture, flexibility, and strength.)

1. Partial Squats

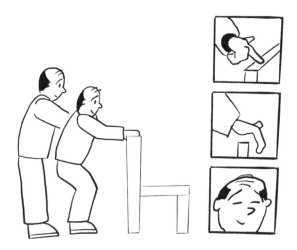

a. Stand 8-12 inches in front of a chair or counter.
b. Hold the chair or counter for support.
c. Slowly lower your body by bending both knees to a position between sitting and standing.
d. Hold the position for 3-5 seconds.
e. Slowly extend both knees to go back to the original position.
f. Perform 10 repetitions for 2-3 sets.

Tip: As you get more comfortable with this exercise, perform the progression of the exercise by first, touching the chair or counter with just your fingertips; second, without touching the chair or counter; and third, closing your eyes without touching the chair or counter.

Why? This exercise will strengthen the muscles of your buttocks, thighs, and legs. By adding the exercise progressions, you are adding a balance training component to a strengthening exercise!

2. Standing Hip Flexion

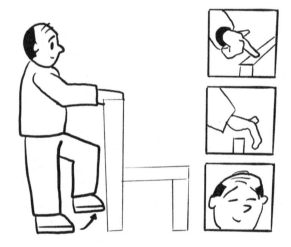

   a. Stand 8-12 inches in front of a chair or counter.
   b. Hold the chair or counter for support.
   c. Bend your hip by slowly bringing your knee up as high as you can.
   d. Hold the position for 3-5 seconds.
   e. Slowly bring your knee down to go back to the original position.
   f. Perform 10 repetitions for 2-3 sets on each side.

Tip: As you get more comfortable with this exercise, perform the progression of the exercise by first, touching the chair or

counter with just your fingertips; second, without touching the chair or counter; and third, closing your eyes without touching the chair or counter.

Why? This exercise will strengthen the muscles in front of your hips. By adding the exercise progressions, you are adding a balance training component to a strengthening exercise!

3. Standing Hip Abduction

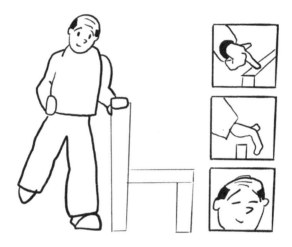

    a. Stand with a chair or counter 8-12 inches on your side.
    b. Hold the chair or counter for support.
    c. While keeping your trunk straight, slowly bring your leg out to the side as far as you can.
    d. Hold the position for 3-5 seconds.
    e. Slowly bring your leg back to the original position.
    f. Perform 10 repetitions for 2-3 sets on each side.

Tip: As you get more comfortable with this exercise, perform the progression of the exercise by first, touching the chair or

counter with just your fingertips; second, without touching the chair or counter; and third, closing your eyes without touching the chair or counter.

Why? This exercise will strengthen the muscles on the side of your hips. By adding the exercise progressions, you are adding a balance training component to a strengthening exercise!

4. Standing Hamstring Curl

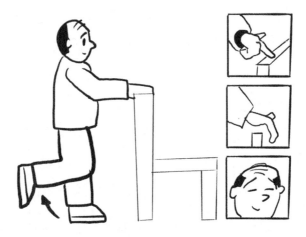

a. Stand 8-12 inches in front of a chair or counter.
b. Hold on to the chair or counter for support.
c. While keeping your trunk straight, slowly bend your knee, bringing your heel up as high as you can.
d. Hold the position for 3-5 seconds.
e. Slowly bring your foot down to go back to the original position.
f. Perform 10 repetitions for 2-3 sets each.

Tip: As you get more comfortable with this exercise, perform the progression of the exercise by first, touching the chair or

counter with just your fingertips; second, without touching the chair or counter; and third, closing your eyes without touching the chair or counter.

Why? This exercise will strengthen the muscles at the back of your thigh. By adding the exercise progressions, you are adding a balance training component to a strengthening exercise!

5. Standing Heel/Toe Raises

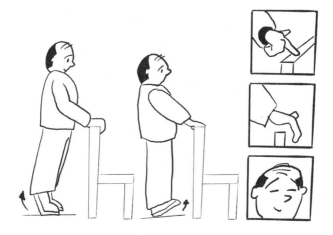

a. Stand 8-12 inches in front of a chair or counter.
b. Hold on to the chair or counter for support.
c. Slowly bring both heels up as high as you can.
d. Hold the position for 3-5 seconds.
e. Slowly bring your heels down to back to their original position.
f. Slowly bring toes up as high as you can.
g. Slowly bring toes back to their original position.
h. Perform 10 repetitions for 2-3 sets.

Tip: As you get more comfortable with this exercise, perform the progression of the exercise by first, touching the chair or counter with just your fingertips; second, without touching the chair or counter; and third, closing your eyes without touching the chair or counter.

Why? This exercise will strengthen the muscles of your leg and foot. By adding the exercise progressions, you are adding a balance training component to a strengthening exercise!

STABILITY EXERCISES
(To improve trunk and posture control.)

1. Forward Reach while Standing on Balance Pad.

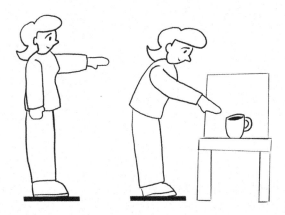

    a. Stand on a balance pad or thick carpet with your feet hip-width apart.

    b. Place an object 15 inches in front of you.

    c. Without moving your feet, reach as far forward as you can toward the object without losing your balance.

d. Return to the original position.

e. Perform 8-10 repetitions with each hand.

Why? This is a progression of the forward reach exercise you performed in the prior level. By standing on a balance pad or thick carpet, you are reducing the stability of your support surface, thereby, challenging your balance even more. This exercise will increase your "margin of stability" by improving your ability to control your trunk and posture.

2. Side Reach while Standing on Balance Pad.

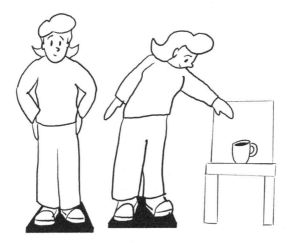

a. Stand on a balance pad or thick carpet with your feet hip-width apart.

b. Place an object 15 inches to your side.

c. Without moving your feet, reach as far as you can toward the object at your side without losing your balance.

d. Return to the original position.

e. Perform 8-10 repetitions on each side.

Why? This is a progression of the side reach exercise you performed in the prior level. By standing on a balance pad or thick carpet, you are reducing the stability of your support surface, thereby, by challenging your balance even more. This exercise will increase your "margin of stability" by improving your ability to control your trunk and posture.

3. Standing Foot Drawings

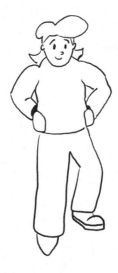

a. Stand with your feet hip-width apart.
b. Shift your weight to one side.
c. Point the opposite foot forward to draw an imaginary square or circle on the floor.
d. Draw 10 imaginary squares or circles on the floor with each foot.

Why? This is a fun exercise to challenge your balance by standing on one stable foot while the other foot is moving. This exercise will improve your agility and weight-shifting abilities during stepping and walking.

4. Standing Ball Rolling

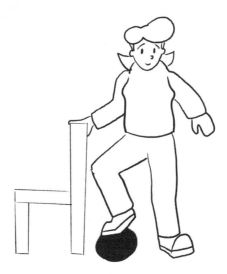

a. Stand with a ball underneath one foot.
b. Hold on to a chair or counter for support.
c. Slowly roll the ball in a circular pattern on the floor.
d. "Draw" 10 circles on the floor with each foot.

Why? Another fun exercise to challenge your balance by standing on one stable foot while the other foot is moving or unsteady. This exercise will improve your weight-shifting abilities and agility during stepping and walking.

5. Standing while Reading a Book

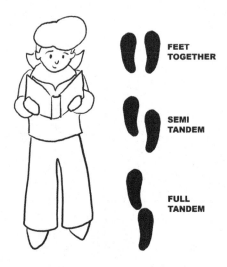

FEET TOGETHER

SEMI TANDEM

FULL TANDEM

a. Stand with your feet hip-width apart.

b. After every paragraph you read in a book, change the position of your feet by following the foot patterns illustrated above.

Why? This is a great way to improve your balance without having to always look down at your feet.

TRANSITION EXERCISES
(To prevent balance loss when changing positions.)

1. Step-Ups

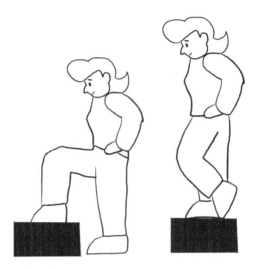

    a. Stand 6-8 inches in front of a step or step stool.
    b. Start with one foot up on the step or step stool.
    c. Step up by bringing your other foot up on the step or step stool.
    d. Slowly step back down by bringing one foot back to the floor.
    e. Perform 10 repetitions on each side.

Why? Some falls happen during the transition movement of stepping up or down. This exercise will not only strengthen the muscles in your buttocks, hips, thighs, and legs, it will also train your brain and body to anticipate the postural changes required to step up or step down without losing your balance.

2. Side Step-ups

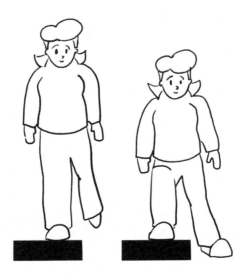

a. Stand on the side of a step or step stool.
b. Start with one foot up on the step or step stool.
c. Keeping your trunk straight, step up by bringing your other foot up on the step or step stool.
d. Slowly step back down by bringing one foot back to the floor.
e. Perform 10 repetitions on each side.

Why? This exercise will strengthen the muscles in your buttocks, the side of your hips, thighs, and legs. This will also strengthen your postural muscles that are required to keep your pelvis even and your posture erect during standing and walking.

6. One-Legged Stance

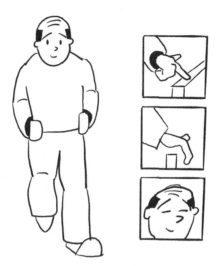

a. Stand with both feet hip-width apart.
b. Hold on to a chair or counter for support.
c. Bring one foot off the floor and hold the position for 3-5 seconds.
d. Slowly bring your foot back down to the original position.
e. Perform 10 repetitions on each side.

Tip: As you get more comfortable with this exercise, perform the progression of the exercise by first touching the chair or counter with just your fingertips; second, without touching the chair or counter; and third, closing your eyes without touching the chair or counter.

Why? This exercise will train your brain and body to maintain your balance while standing on one foot. If you think about it, you are standing on one foot each time you swing one leg forward to take a step!

7. Stand on Tiptoes and Reach Overhead

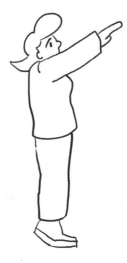

a. Stand with your feet hip-width apart.

b. Shift your weight forward and stand on your toes.

c. Reach up with your hands as high as you can without losing your balance.

d. Hold the position for 3-5 seconds.

e. Bring your hands down to your sides and go back to the original position.

f. Perform 8-10 repetitions.

Why? This exercise simulates the movement and balance required when reaching for objects overhead.

MULTISENSORY TRAINING IN STANDING
(To optimize use and function of sensory systems.)

1. Standing Ball Toss with Eye Tracking

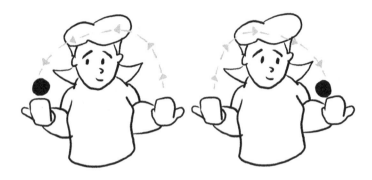

   a. Stand with your feet hip-width apart.
   b. Hold a tennis ball in one hand.
   c. Toss the tennis ball to your other hand, following the ball with your eyes.
   d. Perform 10-12 repetitions.

Why? This exercise will challenge your balance while performing quick body movements with eye tracking. This will improve your reactive and anticipatory postural control responses by improving your reaction speed and coordination.

2. Bouncing/Catching a Ball

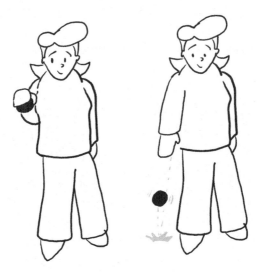

a. Stand with your feet hip-width apart.

b. Hold a tennis ball in one hand.

c. Bounce the tennis ball on the floor and catch it with the same hand.

d. Perform 10-12 repetitions on each hand.

Why? This exercise will challenge your balance while performing quick body movements with eye tracking. This will improve your reactive and anticipatory postural control responses by improving your reaction speed and coordination.

3. Visual-Vestibular Exercises

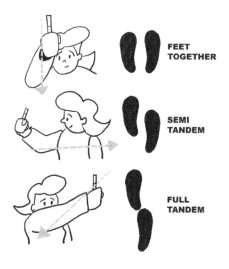

a. Stand with your feet hip-width apart.
b. Holding a pen (or business card) as a target, keep your eyes fixed on target.
c. Slowly move the target up-down, side-to-side, or diagonally.
d. Follow your target with your eyes and head moving in the same direction.
e. Perform 5 repetitions in each direction.

Tip: As you get comfortable with this exercise, change the position of your feet by following the foot patterns illustrated above.

Why? This exercise will sharpen your visual and vestibular functions by improving your visual focus while your head is moving.

STEP TRAINING
(To improve agility, coordination, and reaction time.)

1. **Star Step with Gaze Stabilization**

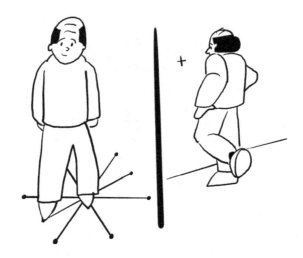

a. Stand in the middle of an imaginary star on the floor.

b. Set your metronome to between 30-60 beats per minute (bpm), depending on your comfort level and reaction time.

c. While looking at an object or target 5-8 feet away from you, follow each beat of the metronome by stepping as far as you can to each point of an imaginary star on the floor.

d. Repeat 2-3 sets of 2 minutes each.

Tip: Take a large step because only with a large step can you effectively catch yourself if you lose your balance.

Why? This exercise will improve your stepping strategy by increasing the accuracy of your foot placement, reaction time, and coordination. By looking at a stationary object or target, you are sharpening your gaze direction and visual acuity during activities involving active head and body movements.

LEVEL 5

MULTISENSORY EXERCISES
(To optimize use and function of sensory systems.)

1. Gaze Stabilization with One Foot on Step

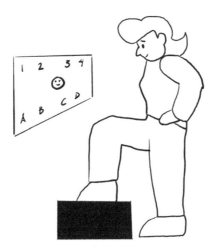

a. Stand with one foot on a step or step stool.
b. Look at a stationary object or target 5-8 feet away from you.
c. Keep your eyes focused on the stationary object or target while moving your head side-to-side or up and down.
d. Perform 15-20 repetitions for 2-3 sets.

Why? This exercise is a progression of the gaze stabilization exercise you did while standing. By placing one foot up on a step or step stool, you are reducing your reliance on an even surface support for balance while emphasizing a stable visual focus.

2. Gaze Stabilization while Marching

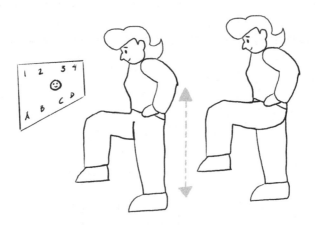

a. Stand with your feet hip-width apart.
b. Look at a stationary object or target 5-8 feet away from you.
c. Start marching in place.
d. While marching in place, keep your eyes focused on the stationary object or target while moving your head side-to-side or up and down.
e. Perform 15-20 repetitions for 2-3 sets.

Why? Marching in place adds a dynamic component that will improve your balance and motion sensitivity while emphasizing a stable visual focus.

3. Gaze Stabilization while Standing on Balance Pad

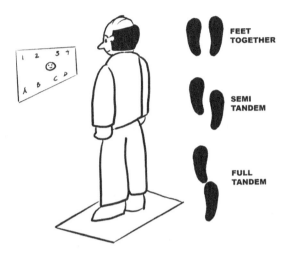

a. Stand on a balance pad or thick carpet with your feet hip-width apart.

b. Look at a stationary object or target 5-8 feet away from you.

c. Keep your eyes focused on the stationary object or target while moving your head side-to-side or up and down.

d. Perform 15-20 repetitions for 2-3 sets.

Tip: As you get comfortable with this exercise, change the position of your feet by following the foot patterns illustrated above.

Why? By standing on a balance pad or thick carpet, you are reducing your reliance on a stable support surface to keep your balance. This exercise emphasizes a stable visual focus, allowing you to keep your balance even when you are standing on a less stable surface.

STABILITY EXERCISES WHILE WALKING
(To improve balance while moving.)

1. Varied Step Length and Walking Speed

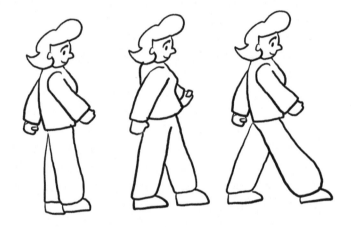

a. Walk across the room and vary your step length by taking small steps, progressing to medium- and large steps.

b. Walk back across the room and vary your walking speed from slow to fast, and from fast to slow pace of walking.

Why? Varying your step length and speed of walking will increase your balance awareness and control so you can adjust appropriately to unexpected challenges to your balance while walking.

2. Walking with Head Nods

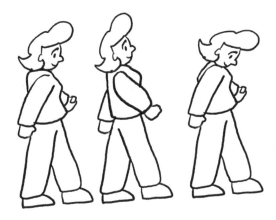

   a. Ensure there are no obstacles in your path.
   b. Start walking while slowly nodding your head up and down.

Why? This exercise will improve your stability during dynamic activities and improve your ability to look up or down without losing your balance.

3. Walking with Head Turns

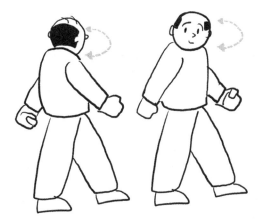

a. Ensure there are no obstacles in your path.
b. Start walking while slowly turning your head from one side to the other.

Why? This exercise will improve your stability during dynamic activities and improve your ability to turn your head while walking without losing your balance.

4. Walk with Pivot Turns

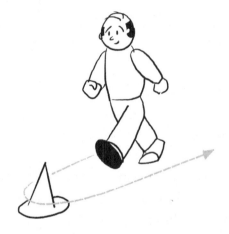

a. Place a cone (or water bottle) across the room.
b. Walk toward the cone (or water bottle) and turn around to head back in the opposite direction.

Why? This exercise will improve your ability to turn during dynamic activities without losing your balance.

5. Braiding

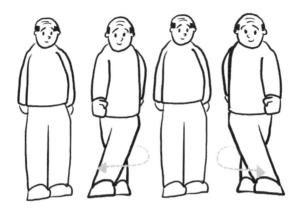

a. Move your left foot directly in front of your right foot.

b. Return to the original position by moving your right foot next to your left foot.

c. Move your right foot directly in front of your left foot.

d. Return to the original position by moving your left foot next to your right foot.

e. Perform 8-10 repetitions.

Why? This exercise will improve your coordination and lateral stability to lower your risk of sideways falls.

6. Backward Steps

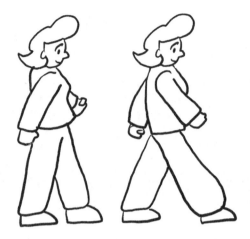

a. Stand with your feet hip-width apart.
b. Practice stepping backward, keeping your feet hip-width apart.

Why? This exercise will improve your coordination and stability to lower your risk of backward falls; i.e., stepping back to sit on a chair.

7. Side Steps

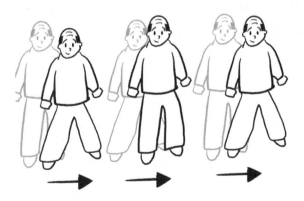

a. Step sideways in one direction.
b. Step sideways in the opposite direction.

Why? This exercise will improve your coordination and agility for lateral stepping activities to lower your risk of sideways falls. This will come in handy during instances requiring you to squeeze through a tight space; i.e., when you are getting to a seat in a theater.

STEP TRAINING
(To improve agility, coordination, and reaction time.)

1. Star Step + Cognitive Task

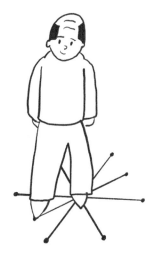

a. Stand in the middle of an imaginary star on the floor.
b. Set your metronome to between 30-60 beats per minute (bpm), depending on your comfort level and reaction time.

c. Follow each beat of the metronome by stepping as far as you can to each point of an imaginary star on the floor.

d. Each time you take a step, concurrently count down by 3's from 100-0 (100, 97, 94, 91...)

e. Repeat 2-3 sets of 2 minutes each.

Tip: Take a large step, as only with a large step can you effectively catch yourself if you lose your balance.

Why? This is a dual-task exercise that will improve your stepping strategy by increasing the accuracy of your foot placement, reaction time, and coordination while performing a concurrent cognitive task.

LEVEL 6

MULTISENSORY TRAINING

(To optimize use and function of sensory systems.)

1. Smooth Pursuit while Standing on Balance Pad

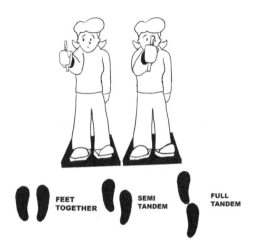

a. Stand on a balance pad or thick carpet with your feet hip-width apart.

b. Hold a pen (or business card) in front of you.

c. Keep your head still while your eyes are focused on the pen.

d. Move the pen (or business card) from side-to-side or up/down, following it with your eyes only.

e. Perform 15-20 repetitions for 2-3 sets.

Tip: As you get comfortable with this exercise, change the position of your feet by following the foot patterns illustrated above.

Why? By standing on a balance pad or thick carpet, you are reducing your surface support and feedback, stimulating increase use of vision for balance.

2. Saccades while Standing on Balance Pad

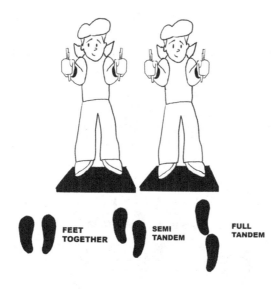

FEET TOGETHER   SEMI TANDEM   FULL TANDEM

a. Stand on a balance pad or thick carpet with your feet hip-width apart.

b. Hold two pens (or business cards) placed about 12 inches apart in front of you.

c. Keep your head still and move your eyes quickly to focus on the pens (or business cards) from side-to-side or up/down.

d. Perform 15-20 repetitions for 2-3 sets.

Tip: As you get comfortable with this exercise, change the position of your feet by following the foot patterns illustrated above.

Why? By standing on a balance pad or thick carpet, you are reducing your surface support and feedback, stimulating increase use of your vision for balance.

3. Gaze Stabilization while Standing on Balance Pad

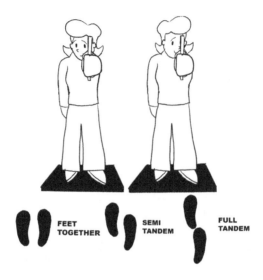

FEET TOGETHER   SEMI TANDEM   FULL TANDEM

   a. Stand on balance pad or thick carpet with your feet hip-width apart.

   b. Hold a pen (or business card) in front of you.

   c. Keep your eyes focused on the pen while moving your head from side-to-side or up and down.

   d. Perform 15-20 repetitions for 2-3 sets.

Tip: As you get comfortable with this exercise, change the position of your feet by following the foot patterns illustrated above.

Why? By standing on a balance pad or thick carpet, you are reducing your surface support and feedback, stimulating increase use of vision for balance.

4. Visual-vestibular Exercise while standing on Balance Pad

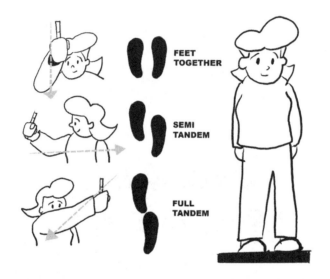

a. Stand with your feet hip-width apart.
b. Holding a pen (or business card) as a target, keep your eyes fixed on the target.
c. Slowly move target up-down, side-to-side, or diagonally.
d. Follow your target with your eyes and head moving in the same direction.
e. Perform 5 repetitions in each direction.

Tip: As you get comfortable with this exercise, change the position of your feet by following the foot patterns illustrated above.

Why? This exercise will sharpen your visual and vestibular functions by improving your visual focus while your head is moving.

STABILITY EXERCISES WHILE WALKING
(To improve your dynamic stability and balance.)

1. Walking with Ball on Plate

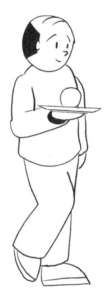

   a. Place a tennis ball on a plastic plate or tray.

   b. Carry the plate or tray across the room without "spilling" the ball off the plate or tray.

Tip: Maintain a safe pace when walking; completion of the task is more important than speed.

Why? This exercise will improve your posture and dynamic stability when carrying objects while walking.

2. Tandem Walking

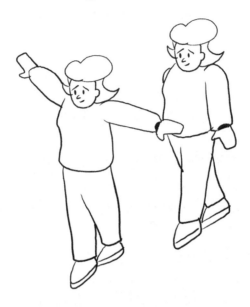

   a. Position one foot directly in front of the other.
   b. Walk an imaginary straight line by alternately placing one foot directly in front of the other.

Why? This exercise will improve your ability to walk through narrow spaces by increasing your lateral stability when moving forward.

3. Figure of 8

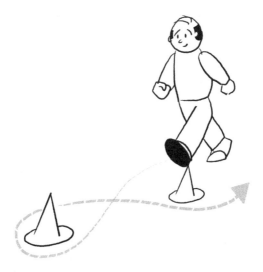

    a. Put two cones (or water bottles) on the floor 4-5 feet apart.

    b. Walk in a direction that creates the shape of the number 8 on the floor.

Tip: Keep a stable base of support by keeping your feet apart when you turn.

Why? This exercise will improve your ability to turn during dynamic activities; i.e., when you need to maneuver through crowds.

4. Stepping Over Obstacles

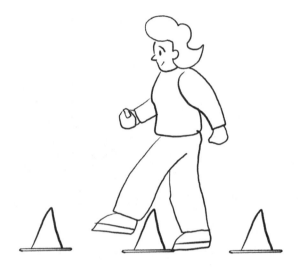

    a. Line up 4-5 cones (or water bottles) on the floor.

    b. Walk up to the cones (or water bottles) and step over them by bending your hip and raising your knee up to clear your foot of the cones without toppling them down.

Why? This exercise will improve your ability to clear your foot off the ground when you walk, decreasing your risk of trips and falls.

5. Picking Up Objects while Walking

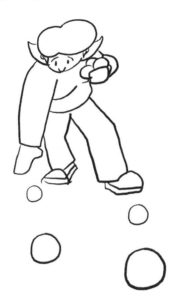

a. Line up several bean bags (or crumpled papers) on the floor across the room.
b. Walk up to the bean bags (or crumpled papers) and pick them off the floor one by one.

Why? This exercise will improve your ability to change your position in space and adjust to changes and obstacles in the environment while keeping your balance.

STEP TRAINING

(To improve agility, coordination, and reaction time.)

1. Star Step + Secondary Motor Task

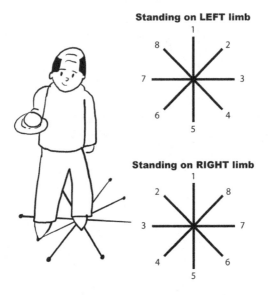

Standing on LEFT limb

Standing on RIGHT limb

a. Stand in the middle of an imaginary star on the floor.

b. Set your metronome to between 30-60 beats per minute (bpm), depending on your comfort level and reaction time.

c. Place a tennis ball on a plastic plate or tray. (Or hold a glass of water.)

d. While holding the plate or tray with the tennis ball (or a glass of water), follow each beat of the metronome by stepping as far as you can to each point of an imaginary star on the floor.

e. Each time you take a step, concurrently count down by 3's from 100-0 (100, 97, 94, 91, etc.)

    f.   Repeat 2-3 sets of 2 minutes each.

Tip: Take a large step because only with a large step can you effectively catch yourself if you lose your balance.

Why? This is a dual-task exercise requiring your attention on two concurrent activities. This exercise will improve your coordination and balance while performing two different tasks at the same time.

EPILOGUE

Facts about Falls

More than **1 out 4** older adults fall each year.
Each year, **2.8 million** older adults are treated in emergency rooms for fall injuries.
More than **95%** of hip fractures are caused by falling.
Falls are the most common cause of **traumatic brain injuries** (TBI).
Falling once **doubles** your chances of falling again.

- https://www.cdc.gov/homeandrecreationalsafety/falls/adultfalls.html
Accessed March 4, 2017

According to the Centers for Disease Control and Prevention (CDC), **every second of every day** in the United States an older adult falls, making falls the number one cause of injuries and deaths from injury among older Americans.[1] Falls present a real risk to the health, independence, and life of older adults.

In this book, you have discovered the many factors that can cause a person to fall. You also have learned about the many different exercises you can do to improve your balance and decrease your risk of falling.

Although, I'll be the first to admit that the information you learned from this book is not a magic bullet that will solve all the falls and balance problems in the world, if it helped you and the next person you shared this book with, you and I have done our share to improve the statistics.

Imagine a life *free* from fear of falling.

Imagine a vibrant and independent life.

Imagine a life of balance.

Join the *BALANCE MOVEment*!

Allow me to re-emphasize: I believe you now have the information that will help solve the growing problem of falling among older adults. Knowledge though, if not applied, is powerless. Let me encourage you to act on the information you now possess:

First, download the free resources I have prepared for you at www.thebookofbalance.com/resources. Even though I wrote **The Book of Balance** to help you figure out the intricacies of balance as easily as possible, it still requires some dedication and effort on your part. The free resources you will download will be a valuable resource as you embark on this very important journey of improving your balance.

Next, share this book with your friends or loved ones. Every successful movement has one thing at its core: effective collaboration. A sage once said, "We all could learn from somebody in our life." Be the person *somebody* in your life learns from. If you and I share the information found in this book, we can make a difference in the life of another human being. Or a million. *A rising tide lifts all boats.*

Finally, I really want you to improve your balance and live a vibrant, fear-free life! I'd like to invite you to share your story or post your picture, along with your "before and after" ABC or TUG score (see Chapter 2) on our Facebook page at Facebook/*BalanceMovement*. Share the improvements in your score and motivate others embarking on the same journey as you. The stories you share will be a boost to the next person looking for a leg-up in their own pursuit of better balance.

In closing, let me thank and congratulate you on investing in your health, balance, and independence.

In over twenty years as a physical therapist, I meet people all the time who wish for better health, but I meet far fewer who, like you, are willing to do something about it.

Let us **redefine** a life of balance.

Sincerely,

Lex Gonzales, PT, DPT

BIBLIOGRAPHY

American Geriatrics Society, British Geriatrics Society, and American Academy of Orthopaedic Surgeons Panel on Falls Prevention Guideline for the prevention of falls in older persons. *J Am Geriatr Soc.* 2001;49(5):664–672.

American Geriatrics Society/British Geriatrics Society clinical practice guideline: prevention of falls in older persons. http://www.medcats.com/FALLS/frameset.htm. Accessed April 3, 2017.

Barnett A, Smith B, Lord SR, Williams M, Baumand A. Community-based group exercise improves balance and reduces falls in at-risk older people: a randomized controlled trial. Age Ageing. 2003;32(4):407–414.

Blake AJ, Morgan K, Bendall MJ, Dal-losso H, et al. Falls by elderly people at home: prevalence and associated risk factors. Age and Ageing 1988;17: 365-372

Chang JT, Ganz DA. Quality indicators for falls and mobility problems in vulnerable elders. *J Am Geriatr Soc.* 2007;55(suppl 2): S327–S334.

Cho, B.L., Scarpace, D., & Alexander, N.B. (2004). Tests of stepping as indicators of mobility, balance, and fall risk in balance-impaired older adults. Journal of the American Geriatrics Society, 52(7), 1168-1173.

Cho SI, An DH, Yoo WG. Effects of recreational exercises on the strength, flexibility, and balance of old-old elderly individuals. J PhysTher Sci. 2014;26(10):1583–1584.

Clemson L, Fiatarone Singh MA, Bundy A, et al. Integration of balance and strength training into daily life activity to reduce rate of falls in older people (the LiFE study): randomized parallel trial. BMJ. 2012;345: e4547.

Dillon CF, Gu Q, Hoffman HJ, Chia-Wen K. Vision, Hearing, Balance, and Sensory Impairment in Americans Aged 70 Years and Over: United States, 1999-2006. Published April 2010. Accessed November 29, 2014. NCHS Data Brief Number 31.

Dorfman M, Herman T, Brozgol M, et al. Dual-task training on a treadmill to improve gait and cognitive function in elderly idiopathic fallers. J Neuro Phys Ther. 2014 Oct;38(4):246-53

Exercise programme aims to cut number of falls across Europe. Nurs Older People. 2014;26(9):7.

Fischer BL, Gleason CE, Gangnon RE, Janczewski J, Shea T, Mahoney JE. Declining cognition and falls: role of risky performance of everyday mobility activities. Phys Ther. 2014;94(3):355–362.

Ganz DA, Bao Y, Shekelle PG, Rubenstein LZ. Will my patient fall? *JAMA*. 2007;297(1):77–86.

Gillespie, LD, Robertson, MC, Gillespie, WH, Sherrington C, Gates S, Clemson LM, Lamb SE. Interventions for preventing falls in older people living in the community. *Cochrane Database of Systematic Reviews* 2012, Issue 9. Art. No.: CD007146. DOI: 10.1002/14651858.CD007146.pub3.

Gillespie LD, Gillespie WJ, Robertson MC, Lamb SE, Cumming RG, Rowe BH. Interventions for preventing falls in elderly people. *Cochrane Database Syst Rev.* 2009;(2):CD000340.

Gillespie LD, Robertson MC, Gillespie WJ, et al. Interventions for preventing falls in older people living in the community. Cochrane Database Syst Rev 2012;9:CD007146

Granacher U, Gollhofer A, Hortobágyi T, Kressig RW, Muehlbauer T. The importance of trunk muscle strength for balance, functional performance, and fall prevention in seniors: a systematic review. Sports Med. 2013;43(7):627–64.

Halvarsson A, Franzen E, Stahle A. Balance training with multi-task exercises improves fall-related self-efficacy, gait, balance performance and physical function in older adults with osteoporosis; a randomized controlled trial. Clin Rehabil. Aug 2014, PMID:25142277

Jalali MM, Gerami, Heidarzadeh A, Soleimani R. Balance performance in older adults and its relationship with falling. Aging Clin Exp Res. 2014 October 7 [Epub ahead of print].

Jefferis BJ, Iliffe S, Kendrick D, et al. How are falls and fear of falling associated with objectively measured physical activity in a cohort of community-dwelling older men? BMC Geriatr. 2014;14(1):114.

Kilby, M.C., Slobounov, S.M., & Newell, K.M. (2014). Aging and the recovery of postural stability from taking a step. Gait & posture, 40(4), 701-706.

Lord SR, Smith ST, Menant JC. Vision and falls in older people: risk factors and intervention strategies. Clin Geriatr Med. 2010;26(4):569–581.

Lord, S.R., Clark, R.D., & Webster, I.W. (1991). Physiological factors associated with falls in an elderly population. Journal of the American Geriatrics Society, 39(12), 1194-1200.

Lord, S.R., Ward, J.A., Williams, P., &Anstey, K.J. (1994). Physiological Factors Associated with Falls in Older Community-Dwelling Women. Journal of the American Geriatrics Society, 42(10), 1110-1117.

Luchies, C.W., Schiffman, J., Richards, L.G., Thompson, M.R., Bazuin, D., &DeYoung, A.J. (2002). Effects of age, step direction, and reaction condition on the ability to step quickly. The Journals of Gerontology Series A: Biological Sciences and Medical Sciences, 57 (4), M246-M249.

Maki, B.E., & McIlroy, W.E. (2006). Control of rapid limb movements for balance recovery: age-related changes and implications for fall prevention. Age and ageing, 35 (suppl 2), ii12-ii18.

Medell, J. L., & Alexander, N. B. (2000). A clinical measure of maximal and rapid stepping in older women. The Journals of Gerontology Series A: Biological Sciences and Medical Sciences, 55(8), M429-M433.

Michael YL, Whitlock EP, Lin JS, Fu R, O'Connor EA, Gold R. Primary care–relevant interventions to prevent falling in older adults: a systematic evidence review for the U.S. Preventive Services Task Force. *Ann Intern Med.* 2010;*153*(12):815-825.

Okubo, Y., Schoene, D., & Lord, S. R. (2016). Step training improves reaction time, gait and balance and reduces falls in older people: a systematic review and meta-analysis. British journal of sports medicine, bjsports-2015.

Orr R, Raymond J, Fiatarone Singh M. Efficacy of progressive resistance training on balance performance in older adults: a systematic review of randomized controlled trials. Sports Med. 2008;38(4):317–343.

Pardasaney PK, Slavin MD, Wagenaar RC, Latham NK, Ni P, Jette AM. Conceptual limitations of balance measures for community-dwelling older adults. Phys Ther. 2013;93(10):1351–1368.

Parry SW, Finch T, Deary V. How should we manage fer of falling in older adults living in the community? BMJ 2013;346: f2933

Rice LA, Ousley C, Sosnoff JJ. A systematic review of risk factors associated with accidental falls, outcome measures and interventions to manage fall risk in non-ambulatory adults. Disabil Rehabil. 2014; 29:1-9

Rogers, M.W., Johnson, M.E., Martinez, K.M., Millie, M.L., & Hedman, L.D. (2003). Step training improves the speed of voluntary step initiation in aging. The Journals of Gerontology Series A: Biological Sciences and Medical Sciences, 58 (1), M46-M51.

Rubenstein L, Josephson K. Falls and their prevention in the elderly people: what does the evidence show? Med Clin N Am 2006;90: 807-824

Rubenstein LZ, Powers CM, MacLean CH. Quality indicators for the management and prevention of falls and mobility problems in vulnerable elders. *Ann Intern Med.* 2001;135(8 pt 2):686–693.

Serra-Rexach JA. Bustamante-Ara N. Hierro Villarán M. González Gil P. Sanz Ibáñez MJ. Blanco Sanz N. Ortega Santamaría V. Gutiérrez Sanz N. Marín Prada AB. Gallardo C. Rodríguez Romo G. Ruiz JR. Lucia A. Short-term, light- to moderate-intensity exercise training improves leg muscle strength in the oldest old: A randomized controlled trial. J Am Geriatr Soc. 2011;59: 594–602.

Shumway-Cook A, Brauer S, Woollacott M. Predicting the probability for falls in community-dwelling older adults using the Timed Up and Go test. Phys Ther 2000; 80:896-903

Shumway-Cook A, Woollacott M. Motor Control Theory and Applications. Williams and Wilkins Baltimore, 1995:323-324

Silsupadol P, Shumway-Cook A, Lugade V, et al. Effects of single-task versus dual-task training on balance performance in older adults: a double blind, randomized controlled trial. Arch Phys Med Rehabil. 2009 Mar;90(3):381-7

T. Hadjistavropoulos, K. Delbaere, T.D. Fitzgerald Reconceptualizing the role of fear of falling and balance confidence in fall risk J Aging Health, 23 (1) (2011), pp. 3-23

Thomas S, Mackintosh S. Use of the theoretical domains framework to develop an intervention to improve physical therapist management of the risk of falls after discharge. Phys Ther. 2014;94(11):1660–1675.

Tinetti ME, Baker DI, McAvay G, et al. A multifactorial intervention to reduce the risk of falling among elderly people living in the community. *N Engl J Med.* 1994;331(13):821–827.

Tromp AM, Pluijm SMF, Smit JH, et al. Fall-risk screening test: a prospective study on predictors for falls in community-dwelling elderly. *Journal of Clinical Epidemiology* 2001;54(8):837–844.

Whitney SL, Wrisley DM, Marchetti GF, Gee MA, Redfern MS, Furman JM. Clinical measurement of sit-to-stand performance in people with balance disorders: validity of data for the Five-Times-Sit-to-Stand test. Phys Ther. 2005;85(10):1034–1045.

Woolley, S. M., Czaja, S. J., & Drury, C. G. (1997). An assessment of falls in elderly men and women. The Journals of Gerontology

Series A: Biological Sciences and Medical Sciences, 52(2), M80-M87.

Zijlstra GA, van Haastregt JC, van Rossum E, et al. Interventions to reduce fear of falling in community-living older people: a systematic review. J Am Geriatr Soc. 2007;55(4):603-615

Made in the USA
Coppell, TX
01 January 2020